ToNiNG
for
teens

ToNiNG
for
teens

The 20-Minute Workout That Makes You Look Good and Feel Great!

JOYCE L. VEDRAL, Ph.D.

WARNER BOOKS

An AOL Time Warner Company

Neither this exercise program nor any other exercise program should be followed without first consulting a health care professional. If you have any special conditions requiring attention, you should consult with your health care professional regularly regarding possible modification of the program contained in this book.

Warner Books, Inc., 1271 Avenue of the Americas, New York, NY 10020

Visit our Web site at www.twbookmark.com.

An AOL Time Warner Company

Printed in the United States of America
First Printing: May 2002
10 9 8 7 6 5 4 3 2 1

ISBN: 0-446-67815-5
LCCN: 200210120

Book design and text composition by Ellen Gleeson
Cover photo by Deborah Beardman

To you, the future generation of young women
who will thankfully be free of endless dieting and
preoccupation with your bodies—now that you know how to
work out the right way! I'm with you all the way.

ACKNOWLEDGMENTS

Thank you to Sandra Bark and Amy Einhorn for your enthusiasm and help with this project, and to my agent, Mel Berger, of the William Morris Agency, for going the extra mile. Thank you to Deborah Boardman for the fine photography and a sense of humor. Thank you to Callie Lefevre, Sara Besnoff, Maureen Bolger, Lauren Szygiel, and Ashley Johnson for doing the workout and the inside and front cover photos. And a special thank you to Jenny Jones and the *Jenny Jones* TV show—it was the e-mails I got from thousands of teens who watch your show that literally forced me to write this book!

CONTENTS

INTRODUCTION   xi

A NOTE TO YOUR PARENTS   xiii

1. YOU CAN GET IN SHAPE!   1
(It's Easier Than You Think
   if You Know What You're Doing)

2. YOU ARE WHAT YOU THINK!   9

3. WORKOUT 101   19

4. WORKOUT DAY ONE: 41
Upper Body

5. WORKOUT DAY TWO: 73
Lower Body

6. TWENTY-NINE MYTHS AND MISTAKES TO AVOID   107

7. EATING FOR FUN AND FITNESS   121

8. EMERGENCY!   139
How to Keep to Your Fitness Plan
No Matter What

9. STAYING IN SHAPE FOR THE REST OF YOUR LIFE   149

RESOURCES   157

INDEX   159

ABOUT THE AUTHOR   167

INTRODUCTION

One of the best ways to ensure health and fitness is a balanced exercise program. As a pediatrician, it is my pleasure to see *Toning for Teens* being published. In it, teens will find a balanced, healthful, safe way to work out with weights so that they will not only get stronger, but acquire balanced musculature as well.

This workout can help remedy the many hours too many of our young adults spend in inactive pursuits. This workout can also help increase the basal metabolism, so that overweight teens will be assisted in weight loss. As they follow this workout, along with a balanced diet such as is found in this book, they will lose excess body fat and eventually arrive at their ideal weight. What's more, we now know that the teen years are crucial in building a bone base, and weight-bearing exercises are the key.

In short, with the permission of your teen's pediatrician, I highly recommend this workout to any young adult.

George M. Azzariti, M.D., F.A.A.P.

Dr. Azzariti is a pediatric specialist who has run the weight control center for pediatric and adolescent patients at Holy Name Hospital for fifteen years. The president and founder of Pedimedica P.A., a group of pediatric practitioners with offices throughout New Jersey, he is a fellow in the American Academy of Pediatrics and has a practice in Fort Lee, New Jersey.

A NOTE TO YOUR PARENTS

Parents, I'm so happy that your daughter has chosen to look at getting in shape in a positive way—and just as overjoyed that you are taking the time to read this note. As a former high school teacher (I taught teens for more than twenty years), I've agonized over how young girls become obsessed with losing weight, and how often I've seen them become emaciated and actually less attractive—the opposite of their goal. I've also felt great compassion for those girls who are overweight and just can't seem to get the weight off—no matter what they do—because they're going about it the wrong way.

As you may already know, I'm not just a former high school teacher. I'm also a *New York Times* best-selling fitness author who for years has done the talk show circuit. My workout books and videos have sold more than three million copies! So for me, writing this book for teens to get in shape is the perfect marriage of my lifelong experiences. But let me explain to you why I chose to do it now.

When I appeared on the *Jenny Jones* TV show to talk about fitness for women, I gave the viewers my e-mail address, thinking that I'd get responses from women of all ages. But instead, I got so many e-mails from teenagers that my e-mail continually shut down. Even though I sat at my desk for ten hours a day, I could not keep up with it. Virtually all of the e-mails were from teenagers—ranging from eleven through nineteen, with the large majority being thirteen to sixteen.

Here are a few in abbreviated form, just so you'll have an idea.

> . . . I want to lose weight on my fat thighs and stomach so I can wear a bikini at the pool and the beach. I've tried dieting and exercising but I don't know what I'm doing. Help!
>
> Sweetie (11 years old)

> I'm 12 years old and weigh 177. How can I get a balanced diet and lose weight? I really need your help because I'm starting junior high school and I want to lose 37 pounds. Please help me, I'm begging you.
>
> Angel (12 years old)

> I'm 13 years old and weigh 160 pounds. My mom weighs only 5 pounds more than me. I was wondering if your exercise program is safe for kids.
>
> Katy (13 years old)

I'm 14 and weigh 185 pounds. I have a loving family but when I get bored I eat and eat. I want to lose 20 pounds by the beginning of school. I'm not taking PE because I have a computer class, so without your help I'll be fatter than usual. Can you help me? I don't know where to start.

Amy (14 years old)

I'm a 15-year-old who is past being overweight. I'm 5'3" and 184. I'm really fed up with diets . . . they don't work. I need to lose weight so I can be healthier, have more energy, and be able to have more fun.

Lilly (15 years old)

I'm 15 and not really overweight by the scale, but I feel fat because my body is so soft. Is there anything you could do to help me?

Tanya (15 years old)

I'm 16 years old and I'm almost as big as my father. I'm sick of living my teenage life with this big fat body. I'm so depressed. My friends say I'm pretty but they are just being nice. My life has become hell because of my weight. What can I do?

Diedre (16 years old)

I'm really insecure about my body. I hate my thighs. I want to wear a bikini but people would make fun of me since I'm 190 pounds and 5 feet 8 inches. Is there a workout I could follow or a diet?

Kim (17 years old)

I'm 18 years old and all my life I've had this dream of joining the national guard. But I can't get in unless I lose the weight and get myself in shape. This weight issue has been a lifelong struggle for me. Do you have a plan that I could follow?

Rita (18 years old)

After reading these letters, you may be thinking, "Isn't it a shame that these poor girls are already worried about their bodies?" You might even be saying, "It's wrong to let society put pressure on them when they are so young." But chances are you're also thinking that it would be good to see our youth being fit and healthy.

That is my reason for writing this book—to see our young women become healthier—and not just physically, but mentally, too! Notice how the girls' sense of self is so affected by their bodies.

My goal is to empower young women by showing them how to take control of their bodies through specific actions. The end result will be a beautifully shaped, strong, healthy body, and also a new mind-set that will carry over into every part of their lives. Self-esteem is improved when people feel empowered.

I want to give young ladies a feeling of control—a sense of being able to make a change by a daily act of discipline—in this case, the simple act of doing a twenty-minute workout four to six times a week, and making informed food choices. As the young ladies do the work, they will begin to see the results in the form of a more attractive body. This isn't a superficial goal, because young women do undergo peer pressure to look a certain way, and it's nice to get that out of the way. But more important, when a young woman sees these changes, she'll make a connection: "By my deciding to do something and then doing it, I can make changes."

When this happens, a change in thinking occurs in other parts of life. It's called the training effect. The discipline learned from working out will remind the teen to force herself to get a term paper done on time, even if she's not in the mood to do it. It will help her study for a test, even if it's the last thing she feels like doing. It will remind her that she can expect and demand better things out of life. It will encourage her to pursue her goals and to believe that she can achieve them. The self-discipline that comes from working out out on a regular basis and seeing the results cannot be measured. You simply cannot put a price on it.

One more point. The workout can head off some very unhealthy attempts to get in shape. I'm reminded of my experience with my own teenage daughter, who was not overweight but was about to become an obsessive dieter because, like most of her friends, she wasn't happy with her body.

My daughter was fourteen years old and looked just fine to me. Then one day I overheard her talking to another girl who in my view was actually underweight. They were planning to go on some fad starvation diet! I took my daughter aside and asked if she and her friend would like to work out with me with weights, explaining to them that when their bodies had feminine muscularity and definition, they would no longer need to lose weight. They would love their bodies.

To my surprise, they agreed and asked if another girl who was indeed overweight could join us. We did a workout exactly like the one in this book. In three months' time, not only had all three girls stopped talking about dieting, they were expressing sympathy for the poor girls who were missing the point and starving themselves to look skinny.

My daughter and her "skinny" friend were now strong, defined, better shaped, and hard as rocks. The overweight girl, who also followed the diet found in this book, had lost fifteen pounds of excess fat and was so happy with her feminine muscularity that she couldn't stop talking about it and showing off her muscles to anybody who would look and listen. After that, this young lady got her mother, who was sixty pounds overweight, into shape!

Perhaps the best-kept secret for teenage girls is working out with weights. I'm here to tell that secret once and for all, and I hope you will help me do it. And by the way, boys can do this workout, too—only they should double the weights since they are naturally more muscular, and they can leave out the hip/butt work since they don't have childbearing hips. Otherwise, it's exactly the same. And I do hope that you too will join your daughter in working out. You can do this workout, or see the resource section for any of my other workouts. And feel free to contact me with any questions or feedback. See page 156 for contact information.

ToNiNG
for
teens

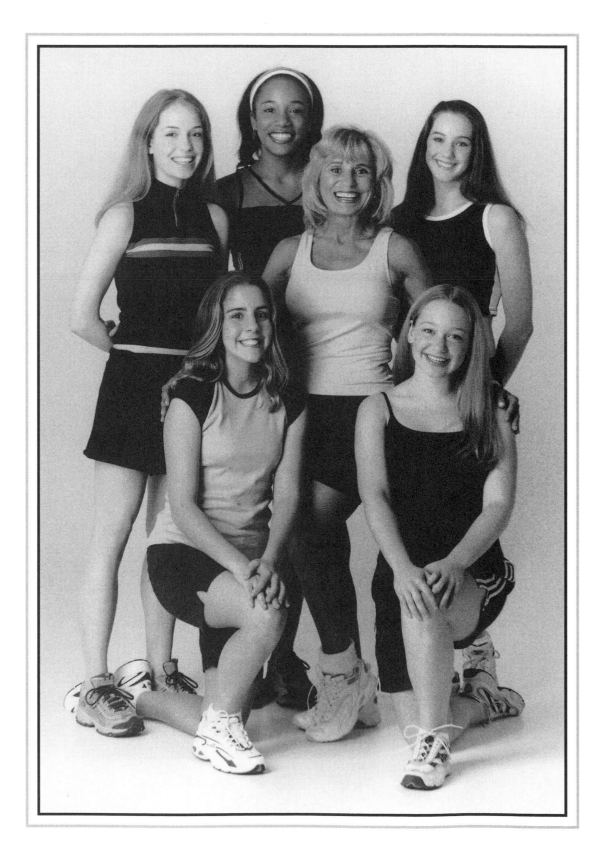

1 YOU CAN GET IN SHAPE!

(IT'S EASIER THAN YOU THINK IF YOU KNOW WHAT YOU'RE DOING)

You've been looking at those other girls and you've been wondering: "Why them and not me—why can't I have a body to die for?" You've been looking in the mirror and thinking, "Yuck. I hate my . . . I can't stand those . . . I must hide my . . ." Well, all of that is about to change. I've worked with thousands of teenagers and adults—getting them into their dream shape—and I'll do it for you.

In this book you will find the foolproof techniques that will not only get you into shape but keep you that way for the rest of your life. And by the way—I'm not just talking about losing weight. I'm talking about having a tight, toned, defined—dare I say it—sexy body, the body of your dreams. By this time next year, you'll be wondering what you were worried about in the first place. But it won't take a year—it will start happening in three weeks, and in twelve weeks you'll look so good you'll wonder—"Could it get any better?"

THE BODY OF YOUR DREAMS

Yes. You'll have the body of your dreams—finally. But what's more important—and this is one of the best things that comes from working out with weights—you'll never wish you had anybody else's body. Why? Because your body will be in its ideal shape—and when that happens, something wonderful happens to the mind. You actually believe in your heart of hearts that you look marvelous. When you look at photos of models and pop stars, instead of wishing you looked like them, you'll think, "I look better than she does." Why? You'll start to notice that some of these teen icons don't even have the shapely, rock-hard muscles you have—and they lack definition. Oh, they may be thin, but you'll realize that many of them are really "flabby skinny"—their shoulders, arms, legs, are not shaped as well as yours. And for those who are rock hard and ripped, you won't care, because so are you!

THE SECRET KEY

Working out with weights is one of the best ways for you to lose weight. Nobody talks about this, which is why I've been dying to write this book. I can no longer bear to watch talk shows and see teens crying out about how fat they are, and then starving themselves down to a skinny fat—and then gaining it all back, becoming even more flabby in the process. The secret key to getting the body of your dreams is not dieting. It is working out and eating right. Yes. Eating for your muscles! You can call that a diet if you want, since the word *diet* really only means "what you eat every day."

So—it's the workout and the eating plan. First and foremost, though, it's the workout, and here's why.

BURN FAT EVEN IN YOUR SLEEP!

Muscle is the only body material that is active twenty-four hours a day. When you put muscle on your body—which takes only nine weeks with this plan—you permanently burn 15 percent more fat twenty-four hours a day, seven days a week, even in your sleep. (Since breathing takes energy, you do burn calories even in your sleep.) While you're doing the workout and following the eating plan, you'll be gaining muscle and losing another body material. Fat! What this means is that you will be changing your body composition.

Muscle takes up less space than fat but weighs more. You may be surprised to see yourself go down a dress size when the scale shows only a slight weight loss. If you're overweight, you'll go down in clothing sizes and your scale weight will keep going down—but the size drop will be faster than the scale shows. Soon you won't care what the scale says. You'll start looking in the mirror, because you'll realize that what you and other people see and feel on your body is in the mirror and in real life—not on the scale. In fact, in time you'll stop weighing yourself altogether, and that would be just fine with me.

WHAT YOU CAN EXPECT FROM THIS WORKOUT

✳ Go down a size approximately every three weeks if you are overweight

✳ Become hard and defined instead of soft and flabby

✳ Increase your metabolism so you can eat more without getting fat

✳ Increase your strength, balance, and stamina and improve in your sport

✳ Improve your posture—look better as you walk, sit, or stand around

✳ Increase your self-discipline—which will carry over into accomplishing dreaded tasks such as term papers, studying for tests, chores, and more

✳ Know and get what you want out of life due to increased self-esteem

MUSCLE VERSUS FAT—AND WHAT KIND OF MUSCLE ARE WE TALKING ABOUT?

Let me explain a little more about muscle and fat—and the kind of muscle you'll be getting with this workout.

Think of muscle as a one-pound dumbbell and fat as a one-pound pillow. Which would be bigger in size? The pillow, of course—much bigger. Which would feel harder to the touch? The dumbbell. So your goal will be to put on muscle and lose fat.

I've been talking a lot about muscles. I don't want to scare you. I'm talking about feminine muscularity—not the bodybuilder kind of muscles that will make you look like a guy. There's no danger of that whatsoever with this workout. To look like a hulk, you would have to work out with weights twenty times heavier than the ones I'm giving you—and you would have to spend hours, not minutes, a day doing it.

Maybe you've seen female bodybuilders on TV and worry that you will look like them. You can put your fears aside. In addition to working out with very heavy weights for hours a day, the ones who look like men take steroids—a male hormone called testosterone. Both men and women naturally produce a certain amount of this hormone, which is needed for normal growth and development, but women who want to get huge muscles ingest a lot of it and suffer side effects such as facial hair, a deepened voice, and rough skin along with big hulky muscles. This will not and cannot happen to you by following the workout in this book. End of story.

WHAT ABOUT DIET?

Now that you understand why working out with weights is the key, does this mean you don't have to diet? If you're not overweight, you don't have to diet. By doing the workout you'll transform your "skinny-fat" body into the body of your dreams. If you are overweight, you should follow the eating plan in this book for your "in-training" body. It's found in chapter 7.

Perhaps the best part of the eating plan is that you get to eat six times a day and never go hungry. In addition to the three meals and three snacks, there are certain foods you can eat anytime, night or day, if you feel like it.

THE SECRET OF THE GIANT SET: WHY THIS WORKOUT WORKS

You'll learn the full details of how to do the workout later in the book, but for now, let me explain why this workout burns maximum fat and at the same time gives amazing definition and feminine muscles. Basically, you're doing what's called a giant set. You do three different exercises for one body part before you take a short fifteen-second rest—and then repeat it two more times with graduating weights. As explained on page 5 with this system, your muscles are not resting long enough to use heavy weights and get big and hulky, but at the same time, they are working in exactly the right way to get rock hard and perfectly sculpted. I learned this secret from champion bodybuilders. It's what they do in the weeks before a contest to get rid of any excess fat and get maximum definition— to hone down the body into its ideal form.

WHY CAN'T AEROBICS OR SPORTS GET YOU THE BODY OF YOUR DREAMS?

We've discussed the beauty of feminine muscularity—but why can't you get that way by doing aerobics or your favorite sport? The answer is quite simple. The only thing you can accomplish with aerobics is to burn overall body fat and to condition your heart and lungs. While these are wonderful accomplishments, they will not reshape your body. The only body shaping you'll get from running is muscular calves. The only leg advantage you'll get from stair-stepping is stronger legs—but your thighs will remain the same shape! The same holds true for any aerobic activity. You get some effect on the body parts that are involved in the aerobics but not sculpting and shaping.

What about sports? If you'd be happy with just pretty legs, then soccer will do it. If you want a nice back and shoulders, then take up swimming. If your only goal is one strong forearm (depending upon whether you're a lefty or a righty), take up tennis. The list goes on.

So you see—there's no way around it. The only way to shape and tone your entire body is to do it body part by body part in a systematic, scientific way, with weights—simple ones at that. Dumbbells. Let me explain.

WHAT WILL YOU NEED TO DO THIS WORKOUT?

The only thing you will need to do this workout are three sets of very inexpensive weights called dumbbells. They are about fifty cents a pound; call your local exercise equipment stores using the yellow pages. They are often called hexes because of the way they are shaped. You'll be starting with two-, three-, and five-pound dumbbells, and since you need two each (one to hold in each hand), it should cost only about ten dollars for the whole set. You will get strong quickly, so if I were you I would also buy three extra sets and put them to the side: eight-, ten-, and twelve-pounders. You can always buy the heavier ones later if you choose to go that far.

If you have a bench, great. You can use a plain flat bench of any kind, or simply use a step as they do in step aerobics. You'll be lying on it, and you only need it for about three exercises. If you don't have any of these, just do those moves on the floor.

ONLY TWENTY MINUTES A DAY: WHY THE TWENTY-MINUTE WORKOUT IS EQUAL TO AN HOUR'S WORTH OF WORK

When most people work out, they use heavy weights, and they rest for about sixty seconds after every set. (A *set* is a group of repetitions of a certain exercise.) In this workout you'll be doing approximately forty-five sets a day. For example, on workout day one, you'll be doing three sets each of three different exercises for five body parts. If you took a whole minute off after each set, you would waste forty-five minutes resting.

With this workout, you only take a fifteen-second rest, and that's only after you do three sets—so when you do the math, you're only resting for a total of three and three-quarter minutes—less than four minutes of wasted resting time. You save more than forty minutes, and in the bargain you burn more fat and get maximum definition—and because you keep it moving, it's impossible to get big hulky muscles. For that you would have to lift heavy weights, and for that you would have to take long rests.

With my method, your twenty-minute workout is worth more than an hour's. And guess what? After you get used to it, you can skip all or most of the rests, and finish up in about fifteen minutes. How about that?

THE TRAINING EFFECT

There are wonderful benefits to this workout. One is that you will become more disciplined and confident. How does this happen? As you get into the habit of working out for twenty minutes a day, you gain control over yourself. Your mind controls your body, and that gives you power. This power carries over into other areas—like getting yourself to do schoolwork or dreaded chores, even if you don't feel like it.

Another thing happens. You begin to feel better about yourself and think more highly of yourself. You begin to respect yourself more than you did before, and your self-esteem improves. When this happens, you learn to expect and demand the best, go after better things in life, and get them! A whole lot of amazing things will happen for you when you let your mind take control of your body.

OTHER BENEFITS

Working out with weights the way you will learn to in this book makes you stronger and more agile—so when you participate in your sport, you'll find that you are better at it. You have more stamina, and you move faster. In addition, your balance is improved, because your overall body musculature is more balanced.

Another wonderful side effect is that you won't feel as stressed out all the time. The workout in and of itself provides a natural high. In fact, many doctors recommend weight training as an antidepressant—and studies show that weight training can take the place of antidepressants for many teenage girls as well as women.

HOW LONG WILL IT TAKE TO SEE RESULTS?

You will see major changes after twelve weeks of working out—but you'll feel something in only one week and see something in three! After a week of working out you will have the sensation of being tighter—more "put together." You'll also start to feel stronger. In three weeks you'll start to see some definition in the shoulder and arm area, and maybe even your upper back. In twelve weeks, if you were overweight, you will have dropped three to four sizes and will be well on your way to the body of your dreams—if you're not there already.

WHY THIS WORKOUT IS FOR YOU EVEN IF YOU'RE NOT OVERWEIGHT

Even if you're not overweight, you might still think you're fat. Why is that? When your body is soft as opposed to hard, you feel fat. The only way to make your muscles tight and toned is to work out with weights. In addition, even though you're not overweight, you may not like the exact shape of your body parts. The only way to achieve your ideal shape for each body part—your thighs, your hips, your buttocks, your shoulders, chest, back, stomach, and calves—is to work each of them individually in a carefully designed program like the one here.

WHAT ABOUT GUYS?

Good news. Guys can do this workout, too—only they can leave out the hip/butt work, since they don't have childbearing hips. Otherwise it's exactly the same. Also, guys will start with higher weights because they naturally have more testosterone and larger, stronger muscles. If you're a guy doing this workout, double the weights listed here and go for it.

BEFORE YOU START

Before you start this workout, I would like you to show the book to your parents and your doctor, and get their approval. Next, I want you to please read through the book and at least skim the exercises so you have a feel for what is coming up. And don't be afraid to write in the book—make your own notes, circle things that seem important. Write your questions in the margin; later you can e-mail me. I answer my e-mail personally (see page 156). You're not in this alone. I'm sticking with you all the way.

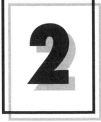

2 YOU ARE WHAT YOU THINK!

The first thing I want you to do is to realize that you are beautiful right now. You are the same adorable, miraculous human being that came from your mother's womb. To make sure you understand this, I want you, right now, to do something that may seem foolish. I want you to go ask your mother for a baby picture of you when you were first born, and some other pictures of you up to your first birthday—even your second birthday. Study these pictures. Look at your smiling face, your eyes, your adorable baby body. You are the same wonderful creation now—only you're evolving into an adult. Along the way, you make a tricky transition where self-esteem is threatened if you don't feel you look "up to par." Well, guess what? Even if you lost weight (and you will) and got your body shaped the way you want (and you will), you would still be struggling with these same issues right now. It's the most normal thing in the world. In fact, if you didn't have some doubts about yourself I would worry.

"I am so ashamed of myself. I look like a fat slob. I wish I could look like those other sexy girls. No wonder the guys hardly notice me." Forget about it. That kind of thinking is going to be a thing of the past. The problem is, most young ladies start to magnify the doubts. Then they take those doubts and form a huge club, and every other minute, they use that club to beat themselves over the head. Stop the music. You're not going to do that anymore. The minute you catch yourself thinking or saying something negative about yourself, I want you to correct it on the spot.

You used to pass a mirror and think, "I'm so fat. I hate my huge thighs. Look at that pot belly." Now, say, "I'm so excited. I'm going to be in training and I'm going to take those sexy thighs and get them into their ideal shape. When I finish following the stomach workout and the eating plan, I'll see the gorgeous abdominal muscles that are now being hidden by the temporary covering—the baby fat." In other words, you're going to get into the habit of reversing the negative thought process.

But what about when other people put you down? Believe it or not, secure people with high self-esteem have no need to put others down, because they're happy with themselves and the world. In fact, secure people are usually kind and helpful to others who are struggling.

Most often it's the people who secretly think little of themselves who insult others. Why? By putting someone down, for that moment, they feel elevated above their "target," and get a moment of relief from feeling like a loser.

By the way, in case you didn't know it, high self-esteem has little to do with looks and body shape. Many beautiful girls with near-perfect figures have low self-esteem, and many not-so-pretty girls who are overweight have high self-esteem. Self-esteem has more to do with your early-childhood and preadolescent and even current experiences with a variety of people close to you.

If anything, if people put you down you should feel sorry for them. They are suffering on a daily basis more than you could imagine. Okay, I know that's asking too much. But at least don't take it personally. Instead, analyze the person as if he or she were a case study. You have the power here. And on the up side, any time you take control of your life and do something positive to make it better, you raise your own self-esteem. So getting in shape will serve a double purpose: It will make you look more pleasing to your own and others eyes, but in addition—and perhaps more important—it will make you have a stronger sense of self. You will believe in yourself and increase your self-esteem.

It's *very* important to realize that the only reason to get in shape is for yourself—to please yourself—and not to please anybody else. You don't have to convince me. I believe you are doing it for you! But if you aren't—if it's because somebody is putting you down or pushing you into it—think about what you need, and decide to do it for yourself.

YOUR IDEAL BODY

There is an ideal body, but it's different for every person. You are going to create your ideal body. When you do that you won't care about how models on TV look. When your body is tight and toned, and you have definition in all the right places, and your shape is symmetrical, you will look and feel so great and so sexy that you will never—and I promise you this—wish you looked like anybody else! It's an amazing thing how this works but it does, every time. When you get into your ideal shape you will secretly think you look better than any model you see on TV. In fact, you'll think, "Hmm. She should really work out . . ."

WHAT WILL HAPPEN ONCE YOU GET IN SHAPE

Another thing to remember is that you're not getting into shape because you think that it will solve all your problems. I want you to realize that losing weight will improve your life in many ways—the biggest being that you will no longer have to think about the way your body looks. You will finally be able to focus your attention on the real issues in life: doing well in school, thinking about your goals, moving toward achieving them, and building positive relationships with family, friends, and the opposite sex.

You will feel and look better. Other good things will happen. Your outlook on life will improve and you'll be physically stronger and able to participate in more sports and fun activities. But there will still be people who reject you, you'll still have problems with your parents, and you'll still go through every other struggle of living in the real world. But you won't be struggling with your body image anymore.

Getting in shape is the beginning of a journey toward discovering your true self.

HOW TO THINK OF YOUR FITNESS AND EATING PLAN

The most exciting thing about this workout and eating plan is that you're "in training." Athletes do it all the time: soccer players, swimmers, boxers, skaters, gymnasts, football players, dancers—they all discipline themselves and work out and eat a certain way because they are in training. You're going to be eating and working out like an athlete! You're constructing a muscular, defined, tight, toned, strong, agile body.

You'll devise a plan where you work out a certain time every day. This discipline will make you feel happy, not deprived. It will empower you. And that power, that training effect, will carry over to other areas of your life. You'll have more discipline when it comes to getting your schoolwork done, keeping promises, and so on.

It's all about using discipline with a goal in mind, and this kind of discipline can make you feel good about yourself and your life. Once you adopt the "I'm in training" attitude, instead of feeling depressed and punished when you find yourself looking at those foods that made you fat in the first place, you'll think: "No. I can't have that. I'm in training." And you'll smile and think of yourself as special and disciplined. When you feel lazy and think about skipping your workout, you'll remember, "I have to do it. I'm in training." And you'll bite the bullet and pick up the weights and start doing it.

THE POWER OF VISUALIZATION AND PRECONDITIONING

Take a before photo. Now draw over it with a Magic Marker, creating the body you want to have. Stand before the mirror in underwear. Mentally picture your body evolving over time into the form you just drew. Now look in the mirror and "tell" your body to get into the shape you have in mind by your target date. (We'll talk about setting a target date in a minute.)

Visualization means to see or "visualize" your goal ahead of time. In other words, you imagine that it has already happened. This makes it happen faster, because your mind is taking the first step. Then your body will follow suit.

Just as you did with the Magic Marker, stand in front of the mirror in your underwear and picture your body evolving into the shape and form you have in mind. As you are working out, imagine the particular body part you are "working" evolving into the shape and form you desire. In other words, as you exercise your stomach, "see" the fat melting away and imagine the tight, muscular, ripped stomach you have in mind.

You can *precondition* yourself by gaining control of your "unconscious" or—to put it another way—"subconscious" mind. This is the part of your mind that goes on automatic and does what you tell it to do if you take the time to give it instructions. For example, as discussed above, if you stand in the mirror and "tell" your body to become reshaped by a certain reasonable date, and you picture your body evolving into that shape, your unconscious mind will begin to cooperate, alerting you when you are going off track, and reminding you to do what is necessary to achieve your goal. In a way, your unconscious mind is like a carefully programmed missile. You can instruct it so that it hits its target right on the money.

To precondition yourself, think ahead and prepare yourself so that when a certain situation comes up, you're ready for it and can control your actions. For instance, you can precondition yourself to resist eating the wrong foods. Let's do a little exercise.

Picture yourself following the eating plan in this book for a few days. Now picture yourself out with your friends at a fast-food restaurant— and they're all ordering thick shakes. Imagine yourself getting ready to do the same but at just that moment, at the thought of the shake, you get a queasy feeling in your stomach—almost as if you were going to vomit. Imagine yourself ordering a no-calorie drink instead.

List the junk foods you will be most tempted by and the situations where you are likely to run into these foods—at home, at school, at your after-school job, out on dates, at parties, and so on. Go through the process above for each food and situation, preconditioning yourself so that when the time comes, you will be one step ahead.

DON'T START THE WORKOUT OR DIET UNTIL YOU DO THIS!

✳ **Psych yourself.** Before you start your new training system, give yourself time to get excited about it and to become mentally ready. I suggest that you read the entire book through, underlining parts that interest you, writing notes in the margin, asking questions (you can e-mail them to me), and so on. In other words, I want you to "own" the book, to make it your own—to put your own personal stamp on it.

✳ **Mark your goal date on the calendar.** This is very important. Don't make it an unrealistic goal. If you are overweight, I would say a size a month is realistic, although you may go down a size every three weeks. Now look at that date and "tell" yourself to get there by that date—remember, your unconscious mind is like a guided missile. It will do what you tell it to do.

✳ **Get your workout equipment and eating plan ready.** Go to the local exercise equipment store and buy three sets of dumbbells. Talk it over with your mom, ask her to cooperate and have the foods in the house that will help you stick to your eating plan.

✳ **Don't tell too many people.** If you have a friend you really trust, you can share your new training plan in the early stages. It's better to wait a few weeks, until your routine is solid. Otherwise you will feel under too much pressure to keep it up—outside pressure. I want all the pressure to come from you! That is a more positive pressure.

MAKE YOUR FITNESS LIFE EASIER

If you know that the moment you get home from school you like to have an snack, have a bowl of precut allowed snacks ready in the refrigerator. This way you won't go straight for the chocolate chip cookies your mom may have in the house for those who aren't dieting. Instead of setting yourself up for failure, create an environment that will nudge you toward success.

PLAN AHEAD FOR PLATEAUS AND STICKING POINTS

After you've been working out for a while, there will come a time when nothing seems to be happening. Don't believe it. At such times, you are actually making a lot of progress—it just isn't showing yet. Think of when you were a child and your parents put a growth chart on the wall. Every year you grew taller, right? But what would happen if your parents measured you every week and one week to the next nothing happened, so they wanted to take you to a specialist because they feared you would never make progress in growing? The doctor would say, "Don't worry. It will happen suddenly."

No one ever sees a child grow, yet all children grow. When does it happen? In their sleep? Who knows? But one day you see it. So it will be with the metamorphosis of your body. It will happen. Relax. Give yourself some breathing room. Keep going even if you see nothing for weeks at a time. Suddenly you'll be shocked to see your muscles and definition.

Don't fall into psychological traps at this time, such as starvation dieting. There are no quick fixes. The best way to get even fatter in the not-so-long run is to starve the weight off your body. Your body is a survival system. When you cut your calories below a thousand, or go on a liquid diet, depriving your body of solid foods, or go on any fad diet that robs your body of balanced eating, your body will lie in wait for the day when you are off guard and force you to eat until you have gained back every ounce of fat you lost—plus a nice amount more in the bargain—to be ready for the next time you try to starve it.

ANGER AND FRUSTRATION CAN BE TOOLS TO HELP YOUR WORKOUT

In life, things make us angry and frustrated. It's just the way it is. You can use that anger and frustration as fuel to power your workout. When you do this, you are, in essence, sublimating your energy. We all do this naturally. You become angry at your parents so you go into your room and punch the pillow. You are frustrated with the mark you got on a test so you tear up the paper. Well, you can take your anger and frustration out on the weights and work out more forcefully than you would if you were in a calm mood. The best part is, the workout will steal away your angry feelings. About five minutes into the workout, you'll feel calm and encouraged—and as a bonus, instead of wasting time and energy kicking doors or fighting with people, you will have accomplished something.

HOW THE WORKOUT HELPS WITH STRESS

Now, here is some more good news. Studies show that working out with weights greatly relieves stress in the very stressful life of teens, and in fact actually lowers blood pressure in those who have problems with it—much more than aerobic workouts do. Why is this so? Weight training engages all of the muscles in your body, and as a result your entire circulatory system is involved, and made more robust. In addition, your arteries, muscle tone, and elasticity improve. This in turn lowers blood pressure.

In a way, working out with weights is a quick-fix therapy session. It calms you down—kind of steals away the agitation. When you work out with weights, you calm down—even if you were planning to stay upset. It's really amazing the way this works.

HOW TO OVERCOME YOUR MIND AND DO THE WORKOUT WHEN . . .

✳ **You're feeling lazy.** You're just plain not in the mood. You'd rather sleep that extra half hour (if you work out in the morning), or watch TV (if you work out after school). You already know how to precondition yourself by visualizing, but what happens when that's not enough? You have to remember your goal—the prize that you're aiming for. Then realize that in order to obtain that prize, the body of your dreams, you have to pay a price. You don't pay the price all at once—you pay it every day in small increments. So even if you're not in the mood, focus hard on how happy you will be when you look the way you want to look and don't have to worry about it anymore. Then hop out of bed or dart into your workout space and get going. You know you'll feel great later. And speaking of later, think of how you'll feel if you don't work out. You'll feel down on yourself. So with that in mind, do it anyway—by an act of will.

✳ **You're depressed and have no energy.** Think of it this way. Whatever is depressing you is not going to get better or change if you don't work out. In fact, it will get better if you *do* work out, because you will feel better five minutes into the workout. Yes. When the endorphins kick in, you'll experience a natural high that will lift you out of your depression. Soon you'll be feeling more energetic and a lot happier. Use your mind and realize that you have power over your body. Even if for the life of you you don't want to, pick up those dumbbells and by an act of will start doing your first repetition. Before you know it you're working out and the whole thing becomes a nonissue.

MAKING PLANS THAT WORK

If you don't make a plan, chances are you won't work out—at least not on a regular basis. So you have to think ahead and decide, "Exactly what time of the day will I work out?"

For many people, the best time is the first thing in the morning, before you even have time to think about it. You can precondition yourself to go straight to your workout area after you hop out of bed, maybe even before you brush your teeth—so you really don't have time to think about it. Before you know it, you're working out and it's over. The workout itself gently wakes you up and you're ready for the day ahead.

But what happens if you oversleep? That's why you must have an alternate plan—a contingency plan. If somehow you miss your morning workout, your plan B is to work out the minute you come home from school. Well, not the minute. You can condition yourself to relax for fifteen minutes—have something to drink and a piece of fruit and then right to the workout area. But once you start, you shouldn't even answer the phone until you are finished. Why? Since this is important to you, you must give it first priority. If you're going to allow yourself to be distracted, you'll weaken your workout. The phone can wait.

Only you know what your life is like. You should think hard and make up a plan. Review the workout schedule possibilities on pages 38–39 and figure out which is best for you. Then write in the times you will work out and stick to it. Make it a priority.

PSYCHING YOURSELF IF YOU'VE SKIPPED SOME WORKOUTS AND ARE TEMPTED TO QUIT

If you fall, just get up and start again. It's that simple. No matter what, the workout is still available, the dumbbells are still waiting for you, the book is still yours. No matter how many times you stopped, you can start again, and this time it will "click." Don't believe the lies you tell yourself. Remember what I said to do with negative thoughts and words: Reverse them. Say, "So you had a setback. A year from now when you're in great shape because you started again, these few days or even weeks won't matter at all."

A year from now you can either be in great shape, the same shape, or worse shape. So don't let a little setback stop you. Just pick up where you left off and keep going.

If you're absent from school for a week, even two weeks, you don't say, "I'll never graduate. I might as well quit." Of course not. You just go back and begin the work. It's the same way with working out. But you're not going to keep having setbacks. You're going to stick with it and go for it because the ideas you're reading in this book are going to sink deep into your mind and give you the power to use your will to achieve your goal.

HOW TO USE YOUR WILL

What does it mean when we say, "Where there's a will there's a way"? It means that if you want something badly enough, somehow you find a way to do it. But how? By using your own power—the power within you to control your own actions.

Let's try to find your will. Think about a time when you decided to do something. Perhaps it was a decision to stop off after school and buy something in the store. You didn't feel like it but you wanted that something, so you forced yourself to do it. It's that simple. The will is the part of you that says, "Do it."

Another time you may have used your will was to do something your parents asked you to do, even though you didn't feel like it, because you knew that if you didn't you would not be allowed to go out. Maybe you used your will to study for a test, and when you got a good mark, you said to yourself, "I did it." Well, it was your will that made you do it.

I'll use one more example. Think of a time when you were too tired to get out of bed—but then a phone call came inviting you to a party or some such fun thing. All of a sudden you had energy. You were able to jump out of bed and get going. Why? You had a motivation. The thought of the fun you were going to have sparked your will.

Well, when it comes to working out, all you have to do is project the fun a little bit into the future. Think about how happy you're going to feel when your body is in great shape, and let that spark your will to make you move—even when you least feel like it.

EVENTUALLY IT BECOMES A HABIT!

The good news is, when it comes to working out, after a while it becomes a habit—like brushing your teeth or taking a shower. After a few months it becomes easier and easier to just do it. In fact, at that point it may become hard not to do it—just the way it's hard not to do other things that are habits. So take comfort. If you can get through the beginning stages, eventually your workout becomes a normal part of your life—a habit. A good habit.

BEWARE OF WILL DESTROYERS

One of the worst things you can do to yourself if you want to have a strong will is to smoke marijuana—or use any mind-altering drugs, for that matter. Studies show that smoking pot causes people to become so laid back that they lose their drive, their motivation, their will.

Why do people smoke marijuana or do drugs of any kind anyway? They want to escape from a problem. They don't want to feel upset. But in fact, that is the worst thing you can do to yourself—to cloud up the problem so that you can't see or feel it. Why? It's the sense of discomfort, the clear knowledge that something isn't right, that sparks your will into action— that motivates you to make something happen, to fix what is wrong.

You get angry. You get riled up. You say to yourself, "I've had it. I'm not taking this anymore." And you use your will to do something about what's bothering you. If you're busy smoking pot or doing any mind-altering drug, though, you kick back and relax. You fool yourself into thinking it isn't all that bad. You do nothing about it. And in the end, you lose more and more control over your life. And let me tell you, in the end, nobody cares about your life as much as you do—not even your parents. In the end it is you who will determine what happens to you.

So why work against yourself and paralyze your will? Concentrate on self-discipline. It builds your will. It alters the course of your life.

THE POWER OF SELF-DISCIPLINE

After all is said and done, the best thing you'll learn from this book is *not* how to get your body in shape—which is a wonderful thing—but how to take control of your life. You'll learn the power of self-discipline. You'll learn how to refuse to give in to your moods, your laziness, your difficult circumstances. You'll learn that you and only you can decide what will and will not happen to your body in a given day. You'll realize that when you use your mind to control your actions, you can in the end control your life—what happens to you in general.

You'll discover that you can overcome the temptation to procrastinate doing schoolwork—writing papers, studying for tests. You'll realize that you can ask for and receive better treatment in relationships with friends and with the opposite sex. You'll learn the importance of keeping appointments, of being on time, and you'll build up a reputation for being reliable. All of this will build your self-esteem. The quality of your life will improve in general.

Think of your workout and fitness plan as training for life. "If I can overcome this, I can overcome anything." And you will—by using your will.

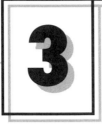

WORKOUT 101

Okay. So you believe me! You're psyched. Now what do you need to know before you start? Not a whole lot, but the little you do have to know will go a very long way, so it's worth taking the time to read this chapter with a pen in hand—and underline anything you think is important.

Let's look at working out as if we were building a house—we'll start from the basics and work our way up.

Let's start with the most basic term of all, *exercise*. What is it? In the weight-training world, an *exercise* is a specific movement for a given muscle, designed to force that muscle to become stronger, denser, and reshaped. For example, the side lateral is a shoulder exercise created to strengthen, define, and sculpt your shoulders into their ideal form.

A *repetition*, or rep, is one complete movement of an exercise, from start, to midpoint, to endpoint. For example, one repetition of the shoulder exercise we talked about above involves raising your arms from the start position, where the dumbbells are held just in front of your body; to the midpoint position, where they are extended outward and upward to approximately shoulder height; and back to the start position again. (See page 51 for a photograph illustrating this exercise.) Now let's talk about a bunch of repetitions.

A *set* is a given number of repetitions of a specific exercise that are performed without a rest. You will do three sets of each exercise. For example, you will do three sets of the side lateral—a shoulder exercise.

A *superset* is a combined set of two exercises for the same body part, or two different body parts, before you take a rest. This is a special technique not used in this workout. We take it a step farther and do the giant set.

A *giant set* is a combined set of three exercises for the same body part, or three different body parts. It saves time to giant-set because you don't have to waste as much time resting—and in the bargain you burn more fat. In this workout you will giant-set all of your exercises—doing three different exercises for the same body part before you take a rest. For example, in your shoulder routine you'll do a side lateral, an alternate front lateral, and an alternate shoulder press. You'll do your first set of twelve repetitions for all three exercises before you take a rest and move on to the next set. (More about this later.) In any case, working in such a manner makes your workout more intense. But what exactly is intensity?

Intensity is the degree of difficulty or challenge of the exercise program you're doing. Intensity can be increased by reducing the rest periods allowed between sets, such as in this workout. It is also increased every time you raise your weights, as you'll do with each set using the pyramid system. (More about that later.) It's also increased every time you increase your overall weights, such as in progression. (Again, more about that later.)

A *rest* is a pause between sets or exercises. The function of a rest is to allow your working muscles time to recover so that they can cope with the next set of exercises. If your goal were to get big muscles—to put on significant muscle mass—you would have to use relatively heavy weights, and you would need rest for about thirty to sixty seconds between each set. The purpose of this workout, however, is to burn maximum fat and make you tight and toned. The only rests you will get will be for fifteen seconds, and not before, as explained above, you have done three sets of the exercise.

A *routine* is the specific combination of exercises that you are asked to do for a certain body part. For example, in this workout your shoulder routine consists of the side lateral, the alternate front lateral, and the alternate shoulder press. Now you're ready to put it all together—you've arrived at your workout.

Your *workout* includes all the exercises you do on a given day. For example, on workout day one you work your chest, shoulders, biceps, and triceps. That's your workout for that day. On workout day two you will do something different, exercising your back, thighs, hips/buttocks, abdominals, and calves.

You can also use the expression *workout* to mean your entire weight-training regimen, including both days. In other words, when someone asks you what workout you're doing, you could say, "I'm doing Toning for Teens."

Now let's talk a little about exactly what you'll be using in your workout, and exactly how your body will react as you do it. First let's deal with what you'll be using—weights.

The word *weight*, as used in reference to your workout, means resistance, or the heaviness of the dumbbell used in a given exercise. You will start with light weights—say, two-, three-, and five-pound dumbbells. But as you get stronger, you will raise your weights. (More about this in a minute.)

What will be happening to your muscles as you do the workout—as you perform the specific reps of each exercise? Your muscles will flex and stretch with each repetition. A muscle is *flexed* when the muscle fibers are shortened as the muscle is squeezed together. For example, your biceps is flexed when you bend your arm and see the biceps muscle bulging. A muscle is *stretched* when the muscle fibers are elongated or lengthened. Your biceps muscle is stretched when you unbend your arm and see the bulge go down—almost disappear.

I'll remind you in the exercise instructions to flex and stretch the muscle as you work out. Be sure to read each exercise instruction before you do the workout. In time you won't have to read it anymore. It will be as natural as breathing.

Speaking of which—don't hold your breath. *Breathe naturally.* When people work out for the first time, they have a tendency to act as if their lives are at stake—they hold their breath! Why do they do this? Nobody is going to kill them. So if you catch yourself falling into this natural beginning habit, just stop yourself by opening your mouth and breathing naturally.

And speaking of breathing, let's talk about oxygen and how we take it in when we work out with this routine, and compare it to how we take it in when we work out aerobically—as when we run, for instance.

The word *aerobic* means "with oxygen." In other words, an aerobic exercise is any exercise you do that can be supported by your body's natural supply of oxygen. You don't have to take a rest for a long time—which can be hours for those highly trained, like long-distance runners.

Technically speaking, an aerobic exercise is any physical fitness activity that uses the larger muscles of the body, and that allows your pulse to reach a state of 60 to 80 percent of its capacity—and stay that way for twelve minutes or longer. (Some authorities insist that in order to achieve an aerobic effect you must work for twenty minutes uninterrupted. More and more exercise specialists, however, are beginning to agree that an aerobic effect can be achieved in even ten minutes.)

If you're interested, you can figure out your maximum pulse rate by subtracting your age from 220. In other words, when doing an aerobic exercise, the highest your pulse should safely go is no more than 220 minus your age. So if you're fifteen, for example, your pulse should not go higher than 205. But our workout isn't exactly aerobic. It's halfway between aerobic and anaerobic. So what is anaerobic?

An *anaerobic* exercise is different from an aerobic exercise in that the activity is too strenuous to be supported by your body's natural supply of oxygen. For example, power lifters have to rest after each lift to recover from the oxygen debt created by the heavy lift. They are forced to stop and catch their breath. Traditionally all weight training was grouped into the "anaerobic" category. With increasing knowledge of exercise physiology, however, fitness experts now realize that the mere appearance of a weight in a workout does not automatically classify that activity as an "anaerobic."

So where does this workout fit in? Since you aren't resting until you have done three sets of three different exercises, it's partially aerobic. In other words, you burn more fat than you would if you had to rest all the time. Yet it's not 100 percent aerobic—if it were, you would never have to rest. But guess what? After you get used to it, you may be able to do the whole thing without resting at all. I do it that way now! Still, this isn't important. What *is* important is that you do the movements correctly, and that you keep raising your weights as you get stronger so that your muscles will keep growing tighter, more shapely, and stronger! And as your muscles become more dense, your metabolism will go up and you will burn more fat 24/7—even in your sleep. We already talked about that in chapter 1.

Now let's talk about the logic of the workout—the method to what may seem like madness. We work a certain way for a very specific reason. For example, we isolate the muscles, use a split routine, use the pyramid system, and use progression.

You are using the principle of *muscle isolation* when you work a given muscle completely and independent of other body parts. In other words, in this workout you completely exercise your chest muscles before moving on to your shoulder routine. You finish all of your shoulder work before moving on to your biceps, and so on.

Muscle isolation is necessary in order to make sure each muscle gets the best possible development and definition. In other words, it's not okay to just do a chest exercise and decide, "Hey, I think I'll do a thigh exercise," and then say, "Hmm. I might as well do a stomach exercise." This is a science. It's not a game! If you want to get in shape you have to do it in a certain way.

Now to more specifics. We don't work the entire body on one workout day—we split it into halves. We use the split routine. What is it and why do we use it?

When you use the *split routine,* you exercise a given number of body parts on workout day one, and a given number of other body parts on workout day two, and so on. The purpose of the split routine is to allow you to work out two days in a row—since muscles need forty-eight hours to recuperate before being challenged again (the only exception to this rule are the abdominal and hip/buttock muscles.)

Back to the science of it all. If you want to get the most accomplished in the least amount of time when you work out with weights, you must do it in a very specific manner. You must use what's called the pyramid system, a system used by all champion bodybuilders for just that reason. What is it?

The *pyramid system* of weight training requires that you add weight to each set with a simultaneous reduction of repetitions until a peak is reached.

Set 1. Twelve repetitions—two-pound dumbbells
Set 2. Ten repetitions—three-pound dumbbells
Set 3. Eight repetitions—five-pound dumbbells

Technically speaking, this is the "modified" pyramid system, but over time it has come to be called the pyramid system. (The "full" or regular pyramid system adds yet two more sets, but we won't be dealing with that here. You can find a whole workout using that system in my book and video *Definition.*)

Now on to one of the most important principles of this workout: progression. What is it? *Progression* refers to periodically adding weight to specific exercises when the current weight is no longer enough of a challenge. For example, in about three weeks you may feel that you are ready to use three-, five-, and eight-pound dumbbells. Two months after that, you may see that you can use five-, eight-, and ten-pound dumbbells, and in another six months, you may be able to advance to eight-, ten-, and twelve-pound dumbbells. And so on. Where does it end? Will you eventually be lifting fifty-, seventy-five-, and one-hundred-pound dumbbells? Of course not. This workout is too intense to allow you to do that. You will reach an eventual "plateau." At this point you will decide whether you are happy with the way your muscles have developed, or you prefer to go heavier and break through the plateau.

So a *plateau* is really a ceiling. Most people reach their weight-training plateau in about a year. If you wanted to break through that plateau, you would have to put on more size by lifting heavier weights and taking longer rests between sets for a while, and then going back to this routine with your new strength. You can find such a workout in my book or video *Weight Training Made Easy.*

Now let's talk about what will be happening to your body—what you will see as you go along in your workout. You will notice an increase in muscle mass, muscularity, and muscle density, definition, and symmetry. All of these combined will be the sum total of your workout: tight, toned, strong, feminine muscularity! A killer body without starving yourself to death.

Muscle mass is the size of a given muscle. You will experience moderate muscle-mass growth as you do this workout.

Muscularity is a comparative term that describes the quantity of muscle on your body as opposed to fat. As you continue to do this workout, and as you follow the eating plan, your muscle-to-fat ratio will increase—that is, you'll have a higher and higher percentage of muscle, and a lower percentage of fat. Your body will burn the extra fat that's under your skin and even the extra fat lining your muscles, so that you'll feel harder to the touch—rock solid! Your muscles will also be dense.

Density is the hardness of a muscle. A muscle is most dense when it has little intramuscular fat—fat marbled throughout the muscle, as I mentioned above. (Think of a piece of steak that is well-marbled with streaks of fat.) This workout will eventually force the fat not only from under your skin, but from the muscle itself.

In addition to density, your body will have overall definition. What does that mean? *Definition* is the clearly delineated lines that separate muscles from each other and divide muscles themselves, making them appear more shapely and attractive. Well-placed definition can also help to give your body a more balanced, symmetrical look. (For example, definition in your upper-back muscles draws attention away from your butt!) Finally, your entire body will have symmetry. You may not be perfect, but you may seem so. How is this?

Total-body *symmetry* refers to the balance and proportion of all the muscles on your body in relation to all the other muscles on your body. This workout will improve your body symmetry in that it will build moderate muscle mass where needed and give ideal definition to your overall musculature.

Some people think, "I hate my thighs and stomach, so that's all I'll exercise." Big mistake! These people will not have total-body symmetry, since their upper body will appear out of balance—not perfectly sculpted, no definition, and soft to the touch. For this reason, it is not a great idea to pick and choose which body parts to exercise.

EQUIPMENT NEEDED FOR THIS WORKOUT

The only equipment you'll need for this workout is three sets of dumbbells and a bench or step—the kind used in step aerobics. You can shove it under the bed when you aren't using it. You will be doing the exercises at home with free weights (dumbbells are considered *free weights* because they can be freely carried about, as opposed to machines that are stationary and bound to the floor).

If you want to use a home gym machine, or do the workout in a gym using machines, you can do that. Just follow the machine alternative at the end of each exercise instruction.

For this workout you will be using dumbbells. But what are they?

A *dumbbell* is a short bar that's usually made of metal—but sometimes plastic—and filled with sand. I recommend the plain old metal ones, usually called hexes because of the shape at the end.

A dumbbell can be held in one hand. It has a permanently fixed ball, or hex-shaped raised section, on either end. Dumbbells also come in "take-apart" sets; you can add weights to either end of them. *Do not get these; they take too long to take apart.* I want you to invest in three separate sets. They cost only about fifty cents a pound if you call exercise equipment stores using the yellow pages. Ask for metal hexes, the least expensive ones they have. For this workout you will need three sets of very light dumbbells: two-, three-, and five-pounders. (Note that whenever I say "a set of . . ." I mean the weight of "each" dumbbell. For example, *a set of two-pound dumbbells* means "two dumbbells, each one weighing two pounds." *A set of three-pound dumbbells* means "two dumbbells of three pounds each." *A set of five-pound dumbbells* means "two dumbbells of five pounds each."

Now to the bench. All you really need is a *flat exercise bench*—a long, narrow padded bench that is parallel to the floor and built especially for exercise. The flat bench can be set on an incline by placing two thick books under its head. If you want to invest in it, you can get a special bench that goes to an incline—but I don't bother with that myself.

A STEP IN PLACE OF A BENCH

A bench is always safest because it's made specifically for many of the exercises described in this workout. If you simply cannot get a bench at this time, however, you can use a step. Note that steps can also be made to incline by using the added pieces provided with the step.

If you don't have a bench or a step, you can do the exercises on the floor.

MUSCLES YOU WILL BE EXERCISING IN THIS WORKOUT

While you're doing the workout, I want you to think about the specific muscle you're exercising, and to picture that muscle losing its excess fat and becoming reshaped into its ideal shape. In order to do this, you will have to know where the muscle is, and how it functions.

Every time you do the workout, I want you to mentally focus on the muscle you're exercising. You can actually double your progress just by focusing and "telling" that muscle to work hard and be reshaped.

Let's talk about the muscles. I'm putting them in the same order you'll find them in the workout: chest, shoulders, biceps and triceps, back, thighs, hips/butt, abdominals, and calves.

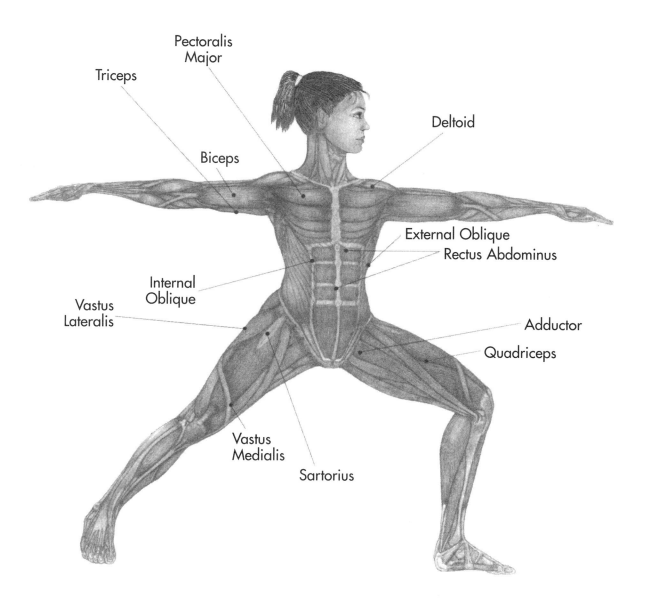

Pectoralis
Major

Triceps

Deltoid

Biceps

External Oblique
Rectus Abdominus

Internal
Oblique

Vastus
Lateralis

Adductor

Quadriceps

Vastus
Medialis

Sartorius

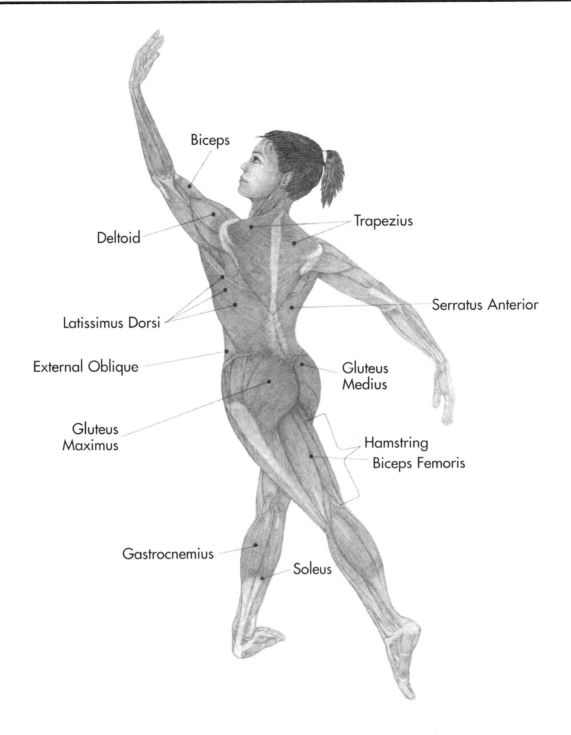

Biceps

Deltoid

Trapezius

Latissimus Dorsi

Serratus Anterior

External Oblique

Gluteus
Medius

Gluteus
Maximus

Hamstring
Biceps Femoris

Gastrocnemius

Soleus

Chest: Pectoralis Major—Pectorals, or "Pecs"

The pectoralis major, a two-headed fan-shaped muscle, lies across the front of your upper chest. It originates at your collarbone and runs along your breastbone to the cartilage connecting your upper ribs to your breastbone. The clavicular head, which is the smaller of the two heads, forms your upper pectoral area, while the larger sternal head forms your lower pectoral area. The pectoral muscles in women are covered by fatty tissue (breasts). To increase breast size, a woman must actually gain fat in this area (and most women do go up a bra size when they put on significant weight). However, breast size can appear to increase if you develop your pectoral muscles—since they're located under the breasts. In addition, exercise gives your chest muscles definition. This definition gives more cleavage.

Your pectoralis muscles function to flex your chest and to pull your upper arm down and across your body.

Shoulder Deltoid

The deltoid is a triangular muscle that looks like an inverted Δ, the Greek letter *delta* (hence the name *deltoid*). It consists of three parts, which can function independently or as a group: the anterior (front) deltoid, the medial (middle or side) deltoid, and the posterior (rear) deltoid.

Your entire deltoid muscle originates in the upper area of your shoulder blade, where it joins your collarbone. The three parts of the muscle weave together and are attached on the bone of your upper arm. One angle drapes over your shoulder area, another points down your arm, weaving around the front of that arm, and the third drapes down the back of your arm.

The anterior deltoid cooperates with your pectoral muscles to lift your arm and move it forward. The medial deltoid helps lift your arm sideways; the posterior deltoid works in conjunction with the latissimus dorsi (see page 29) to extend your arm backward.

Biceps

The biceps is a two-headed muscle (hence the name *biceps*) with one short head and one long head. Both heads originate on the cavity of your shoulder blade where your upper armbone inserts into your shoulder. The two heads join to form a "hump" about a third of the way down your arm. The other end of your biceps is attached to the bones of your fore-arm by one connecting tendon.

Your biceps works to twist your hand and to flex your arm.

Triceps

The triceps is a three-headed muscle (that's why we call it *triceps*). This muscle becomes flabby in older women—because it's one of the least used muscles—unless of course you work out. Your triceps is located on the underside of your arm, just opposite your biceps muscle.

One of the three heads of this muscle attaches to your shoulder blade, while the other two heads originate from the back side of your upper arm and insert at your elbow. The longer head does the work of pulling your arm back once it has been moved away from your body, while the other two heads, together with the longer head, work to extend your arm and forearm.

Back: Latissimus Dorsi and Trapezius, or "Traps"

The latissimus dorsi originate along your spinal column in the middle of your back and run upward and sideways to your shoulders, inserting in the front of your upper arm. These muscles work to pull your shoulder back and downward and your arm toward your body.

These muscles are quite beautiful when developed, because they give your back a V-shaped look that in turn helps make your waist and hips look smaller.

Your trapezius muscle is triangular. It originates along your spine and runs from the back of your neck to the middle of your back. The upper fibers of your trapezius, or traps, are attached to your collarbone and show visible outward development in your neck/shoulder area, but there is more to this muscle than meets the eye. Actually, a large part of your traps are hidden. They really descend all the way down to your lower spine.

Front, Inner, and Back Thigh: Quadriceps, Sartorius, Adductor, and Biceps Femoris, or Hamstrings

The quadriceps, or front thigh muscle, consists of four muscles. (That's why they're called *quadriceps*.) The muscles run along your thigh and end at your kneecap. The four quadriceps muscles are: the rectus femoris, which originates on the front of your hipbone; and the vasti, which are three muscles grouped together: the vastus lateralis, the vastus medialis, and the vastus intermedius, which originate on your thighbone.

The entire quadriceps group works to extend your lovely leg.

The sartorius muscle runs along your inner thigh, from your hipbone to the inside of your knee. It is the longest muscle in your body. Its job is to rotate your thigh.

The adductor muscles are also located on your inner thigh. This muscle group originates from your lower pelvic area on your pubis bone and rises to the shaft of your thighbone, where it is inserted. This muscle group works in cooperation with other inner-thigh muscles to flex, rotate, and pull your legs together from a wide stance.

The hamstring (biceps femoris) muscle group is located on your back thigh. It consists of two muscle groups—the semimembranosus and the semitendinosus. They originate in the bony area of your pelvis and end along the back of your knee joint. This muscle group works to bend your knee.

Hips/Buttocks: Gluteus Maximum, Gluteus Medius, and Gluteus Minimus

The gluteus maximus, as you might imagine from the name, is the largest of your gluteus muscles. It originates from the iliac crest of your thighbone and runs down to your tailbone. It works to extend and rotate your thigh when extreme force is needed—for example, when you climb stairs.

The gluteus medius is located just beneath your gluteus maximus. It works to raise your leg out to the side and to balance your hips when you shift your weight from one foot to the other.

The gluteus minimus originates on the iliac crest of your hipbone and does the same work as your gluteus medius.

Abdominals: Rectus Abdominus, External Obliques, and Internal Obliques

Your abdominal muscle is called the rectus abdominus. It is a very strong, long muscle that is segmented. Because of its segmentation, when it's well developed, it appears "ripped." Well-developed abs are also known as "beer can abs." These muscles originate from your fifth through seventh ribs and run vertically across your abdominal wall. They work to pull your upper body toward your lower body when you sit up from a lying-down position.

In reality, the rectus abdominus isn't separated into upper and lower sections. It's one long muscle, but because it's necessary to isolate the upper from the lower areas for workout concentration, most people think of abdominals as being two separate entities: "upper abdominals" and "lower abdominals."

The external oblique muscles begin at the side of your lower ribs and run diagonally to your rectus abdominus muscle. Your obliques are attached to the sheath of fibrous tissue that surrounds your rectus abdominus. Your obliques work with other muscles to rotate and flex your torso.

Your internal oblique muscles run at right angles to your external obliques and beneath them. It is this angle that forms your waistline, and determines how big or small your waist is.

Calf: Gastrocnemius and Soleus

The gastrocnemius is a two-headed muscle that connects the middle of your lower leg and ties in with your Achilles tendon. The point where the two muscles tie together forms your calf.

Your gastrocnemius muscle works in opposition to the extensor muscles of your lower leg, which pull your foot upward. It also works with other muscles to bend your knee and flex your foot downward.

The soleus muscle originates on the back of your tibia and head of your fibula bones. It lies just beneath your gastrocnemius muscle, but does not pass your knee joint; it works only to flex your foot downward and cannot help bend your knee.

BREAKING IN GENTLY

No matter how tempted you are, do not try to do the entire workout with weights when you first start out. Use this plan to get your body ready.

Week 1. Do the entire workout without weights—just the movements.
Week 2. Do only the first set of exercises with weights. Do the other two without weights.
Week 3. Do only your first and second sets of exercises with weights. Do your third set without weights.
Week 4. Do all three sets with weights. You're ready for the full program.

STRETCHING

The first light set of each exercise serves as a natural stretch. If you have a favorite set of stretches, however, there's no harm in doing them, as long as you don't mind investing the extra time.

DON'T BE DISCOURAGED IF YOU CAN'T DO ALL THE REPS EVEN AFTER A FEW WEEKS

Most people can't do all the reps for certain body parts for a while. For example, it may take a few weeks or even months to build up to the full fifteen repetitions of each abdominal exercise—and you'll be doing five exercises for abs! Since you're giant-setting abdominals, you will actually be doing seventy-five reps before you stop and take a fifteen-second rest.

With this in mind, don't worry if you can only do a few reps of each exercise in the beginning. A good idea is to try to add two reps a week. For example, start by trying to do only three reps of each abdominal exercise in the beginning. If you add two reps a week, in six weeks you'll be doing the full plan.

TAKING FULL ADVANTAGE OF THE EXERCISE INSTRUCTIONS

Your exercise instructions tell you everything you need to know about doing the exercises safely and, at the same time, productively—that is, to get into your best possible shape. Read what the exercise does and which muscle it exercises. Locate that muscle on your anatomy photo—and on your own body. While you're working out, mentally focus on that muscle.

The next item in the exercise instructions is "stance." This is your starting position. Read carefully. Get into that exact position. Look at the photo to be sure. Then you'll come to "movement." Again, before you start, read the instruction carefully. Note where to flex and where to stretch. Follow the actions exactly as written.

Before you even start, you should read the "tips" section so you don't make common mistakes such as rocking or swinging or holding your breath. Stay one step ahead—I'll help you avoid bad habits.

Next, read the "machines, etc." section. I suggest machines you can use (in case you want to do this workout in a health club or gym) and also mention other dumbbell and barbell alternatives in case you want to vary your workout or add more exercises for a more intense workout.

If you do use machines, keep in mind that most exercise machines have only ten-pound weight gradations—so you will probably have to use the lowest weight for all three sets until you get strong enough to pyramid the weights upward for the second and third sets.

You will be happy to see that I have spelled everything out, telling you what exercises to giant-set together, what weights to use, how many reps to do, and so on. This is going to be easier than you think.

HOW FAST SHOULD YOU MOVE?

In the beginning stages, the learning stages, you'll naturally move slowly because you'll have one eye on the instructions. But as you get used to it, you'll find yourself getting up to speed. Before you know it you'll be finishing your workout in less than twenty minutes!

How fast should you go? Not in slow motion, that's for sure. Go at your own natural pace, but keep it moving. I suggest you look at one of my videos if you can't figure out a pace. (You can find a list of my videos at my Web site: www.joycevedral.com.)

HOW TO DO THE TONING FOR TEENS WORKOUT

As mentioned before, this entire workout uses the system of the giant set. This means you do three or more exercises before you take a rest. In a "normal" weight-training workout, you would rest after each set.

Reminder: We are doing it this way because we mean business. We want to save time, get more definition, burn more fat, and get in shape three times faster than "normal."

Workout Day One

Let's talk about how to do the workout, using the chest as an example. Your three chest exercises are:

1. Flat press
2. Flat flye
3. Cross-bench pullover

For the sake of simplicity, I will assume you are starting out with two-, three-, and five-pound dumbbells.

Here's how you do it.

Set 1. Two-pound dumbbells. Twelve repetitions for each of the three chest exercises—no rest between sets. Then take a fifteen-second rest before you begin set 2.
Set 2. Three-pound dumbbells. Ten repetitions for each of the three chest exercises—no rest. Then take a fifteen-second rest and begin set 3.
Set 3. Five-pound dumbbells. Eight repetitions for each of the three chest exercises, no rest. Then take a fifteen-second rest and begin your next body part, your shoulder routine.

Keep going that way. Next do your shoulders, your biceps, then your triceps, then your back. Then you're finished for the day.

Let me spell it out for you another way, to make sure you fully understand. Using the above example, you pick up your two-pound dumbbells and you do twelve repetitions of the flat press, then without resting do twelve repetitions of the flat flye, and still without resting do twelve repetitions of the cross-bench pullover.

Now rest only fifteen seconds and pick up your three-pound dumbbells. Do only ten repetitions of your flat press, ten repetitions of your flat flye, and ten repetitions of your cross-bench pullover, all without resting. Now you rest for fifteen seconds.

Finally, you pick up your heaviest weight, your five-pound dumbbells. You do eight repetitions of your flat press, eight repetitions of your flat flye, and eight repetitions of your cross-bench pullover.

You rest fifteen seconds and work exactly the same way for all the other body parts (shoulders, biceps, triceps, and back) in workout day one. At this point you will have finished your entire workout day one routine.

Workout Day Two

Things are a little different in workout day two. For one thing, you're doing more exercises for three of the body parts—five instead of three. Why? These body parts are thighs, hips/buttocks, and abdominals. They're usually more troublesome on most women, and need a little extra work.

The first body part you will exercise on workout day two is thighs. You will be doing:

1. Squat
2. Lunge
3. Leg curl
4. Front squat
5. Hack squat

Using your two-pound dumbbells you will do twelve repetitions of the squat, then without resting twelve repetitions of the lunge, and without resting twelve repetitions of the leg curl, and still without resting twelve repetitions of the front squat, and finally—still without resting—twelve repetitions of the hack squat. Now you rest for fifteen seconds and repeat the above, doing ten repetitions each with the three-pound dumbbell, and for a third and final time, doing eight repetitions for each exercise with the five-pound dumbbell.

For your next two body parts, hips/buttocks and abdominals, the picture changes. You don't pyramid the weights, because there are no weights to pyramid. To make up for the fact that you aren't using weights, you will do fifteen repetitions of each exercise for all three sets. Here's how it looks using your hip/buttock routine as the example. You will be doing:

1. Lower butt side kick
2. Lower butt curl
3. Lying butt lift
4. Floor feather kick-up
5. Straight-leg kick-up

Here's how you do it.

Set 1. Fifteen repetitions of each of the five hip/buttock exercises—no rest between sets. Then take a fifteen-second rest before you begin set 2.

Set 2. Fifteen repetitions of each of the five hip/buttock exercises—no rest between sets. Then take a fifteen-second rest before you begin set 3.

Set 3. Fifteen repetitions of each of the five hip/buttock exercises—no rest between sets. Then take a fifteen-second rest before you begin your abdominal exercises.

Keep going this way for abdominals, which also have five exercises and do not use weights.

Finally we come to the last body part for workout day two, the calves. Luckily, these are the easiest of all body parts to exercise. For the calves, you return to the pyramid system. Your calf exercises are:

1. The standing-straight toe calf raise
2. The standing-angled-out toe calf raise
3. The standing-angled-in toe calf raise

Here's how you do it.

Set 1. Two-pound dumbbells. Twelve repetitions of each of the three calf exercises—no rest between sets. Then take a fifteen-second rest before you begin set 2.
Set 2. Three-pound dumbbells. Ten repetitions of each of the three calf exercises—no rest. Then take a fifteen-second rest and begin set 3.
Set 3. Five-pound dumbbells. Eight repetitions of each of the three calf exercises.

You are finished with workout day two. You are a champion.

RAISING YOUR WEIGHTS AS YOU GET STRONGER

You may need to start even lighter than the weights used in the demonstration above, and in the exercise instructions. For example, you may need to use one-, two-, and three-pound dumbbells to begin with. On the other hand, you may be able to start with two-, three-, and five-pounders. You should buy all four sets so that as you try the workout, you can see what you can handle. Regardless, in a short period of time you will be raising your weights. If it were me, I would get six sets of weights to begin with—one-, two-, three-, five-, eight-, and ten-pounders. More about that in a minute.

If you start with very light weights—one-, two-, and three-pound dumbbells, for example—in a week or two from the day you are on the full routine you may be strong enough to raise your weights. In any case, you will eventually raise them. Don't push it—but then again, don't hold yourself back. When the weights feel too easy—when you know you could get many more reps than you're being asked to do with the weights—it's time to raise the weights. Never add reps. If you're strong enough to add reps, it's time to raise your weights.

Here's a chart that shows how to raise your weights using the pyramid system as required by this workout:

LOWEST BEGINNING WEIGHTS
Set 1. One-pound dumbbells
Set 2. Two-pound dumbbells
Set 3. Three-pound dumbbells

RAISING WEIGHTS THE FIRST TIME
Set 1. Two-pound dumbbells
Set 2. Three-pound dumbbells
Set 3. Five-pound dumbbells

RAISING WEIGHTS THE SECOND TIME
Set 1. Three-pound dumbbells
Set 2. Five-pound dumbbells
Set 3. Eight-pound dumbbells

RAISING WEIGHTS THE THIRD TIME
Set 1. Five-pound dumbbells
Set 2. Eight-pound dumbbells
Set 3. Ten-pound dumbbells

RAISING WEIGHTS THE FOURTH TIME
Set 1. Eight-pound dumbbells
Set 2. Ten-pound dumbbells
Set 3. Twelve-pound dumbbells

RAISING WEIGHTS THE FIFTH TIME
Set 1. Ten-pound dumbbells
Set 2. Twelve-pound dumbbells
Set 3. Fifteen-pound dumbbells

RAISING WEIGHTS THE SIXTH TIME
Set 1. Ten-pound dumbbells
Set 2. Fifteen-pound dumbbells
Set 3. Twenty-pound dumbbells

RAISING WEIGHTS THE SEVENTH TIME
Set 1. Twelve-pound dumbbells
Set 2. Fifteen-pound dumbbells
Set 3. Twenty-pound dumbbells

How high will you eventually raise them? I stopped at ten, fifteen, and twenty pounds. You can decide where you want to stop. Just look at your body in the mirror and see if you're happy with the way you look. You may be quite satisfied with ten pounds as your highest weight.

IS IT OKAY TO USE DIFFERENT WEIGHTS FOR DIFFERENT EXERCISES?

Yes, but not right away. Why? In the beginning it will be too confusing, so you should wait until you are really comfortable with the program. When you start out, you'll notice that some body parts are stronger than others, but I still want you to use the same weights throughout the workout. After a few weeks, you'll find that you simply can't stand doing, say, your chest—which has stronger, larger muscles—with such light weights, even though your shoulders may still be too weak to raise those same weights. This makes sense, so don't be concerned. In time, you will absolutely raise the weights for even the weaker body parts—and when you feel like you really understand the workout, you can experiment with alternating the weights. But give your body time. It will happen in due course.

WORKOUT PLANS

You can work out four to six days a week with weights. If you do aerobics, you can do them three to six days a week, whether or not you work with weights. Aerobics don't get in the way of weights.

Although the real calendar begins on Sunday, most people think of Monday as the first day of their week so I'm starting the calendars you see below with Monday as the first day of the week. Your four-day workout schedule may look something like this:

Monday	Tuesday	Wednesday	Thursday	Friday	Saturday	Sunday
Upper	Lower		Upper	Lower		

Or it may look something like this:

Monday	Tuesday	Wednesday	Thursday	Friday	Saturday	Sunday
Upper	Lower	Upper	Lower			

Or you might try:

Monday	Tuesday	Wednesday	Thursday	Friday	Saturday	Sunday
	Upper		Lower	Upper	Lower	

Here's a sample calendar for *five* days a week:

Monday	Tuesday	Wednesday	Thursday	Friday	Saturday	Sunday
Upper	Lower	Upper	Lower	Upper		

For *six* days a week:

Monday	Tuesday	Wednesday	Thursday	Friday	Saturday	Sunday
Upper	Lower	Upper	Lower	Upper	Lower	

In other words, never work the same body parts two days in a row! Whatever you worked last time—do the other half the next time. It's that simple.

Okay. Now you're armed and dangerous. It's time to begin your workout!

WORKOUT DAY ONE:

UPPER BODY

Now you're ready to get down to business. In this chapter you'll exercise your upper body: chest, shoulders, biceps, triceps, and back. You'll be doing this workout every other time you work out. You'll be doing three exercises per body part, with the option of doing two more.

You will be working in a very special way so as to burn the maximum amount of fat, get the most definition, and get into shape the fastest possible way! In other words, you'll be doing giant sets, as we discussed in chapter 3.

You'll notice that you're doing chest first, then shoulders, then biceps, then triceps, then back. Why this order? Well, the psychology is to alternate between strong and weak muscles. You start out with a very strong body part, the chest—so you will feel empowered. Then you do a weaker body part, the shoulders—but you'll be able to cope with that because you just did your chest. Now just when you may be thinking, "Wow I'm so weak," you do another strong body part, the biceps. Then you do your weaker triceps. You finish with the strong and easy back—which is also great because you look forward to it as a reward. It's also relaxing because your back stretches out as you work out, and that makes your entire body feel relaxed—something like getting a back massage.

Let's get busy. Review the section of chapter 3 called "How to Do the Toning for Teens Workout," and then simply follow the photographs and exercise instructions. Before you know it you won't even need this book.

CHEST ROUTINE

1. FLAT PRESS

This exercise develops, shapes, strengthens, and defines the entire chest/breast (pectoral) area, and helps give the look of cleavage to the breast area. There are fringe benefits for the upper arms, forearms, wrists, shoulders, and shoulder joints.

Stance: Lie on a flat exercise bench with a dumbbell in each hand, palms facing away from your body, with the inner edge of each dumbbell touching the outer edges of your upper chest/shoulder area. Bend your knees and place the soles of your feet flat on the bench to prevent your back from arching. (Your back should be flat to the bench.)

Movement: Flexing your chest muscles as you go, raise the dumbbells above your chest until your arms are fully extended, but don't lock your elbows. Without resting, return to the start position and feel the stretch in your chest muscles. Repeat the movement until you have completed your set. Without resting, move to your next chest exercise, the flat flye.

Tips: The dumbbells should be in line with your upper chest in the fully extended position. Remember to fully extend your elbows downward in the down position. Don't cheat yourself by doing half movements. Don't hold your breath. Breathe naturally.

Machines, Etc.: You may use the lying bench press machine to do this exercise, or you can use a barbell and a bench press station. You can do this on an incline bench with dumbbells or a barbell.

SETS, REPETITIONS, WEIGHTS:

Set 1. Light: 12 reps flat press + 12 reps flat flye + 12 reps cross-bench pullover. Rest 15 seconds.

Set 2. Middle: 10 reps flat press + 10 reps flat flye + 10 reps cross-bench pullover. Rest 15 seconds.

Set 3. Heaviest: 8 reps flat press + 8 reps flat flye + 8 reps cross-bench pullover. Rest 15 seconds.

Reminder: See pages 36–37 for tips on heaviness of weights and raising weights.

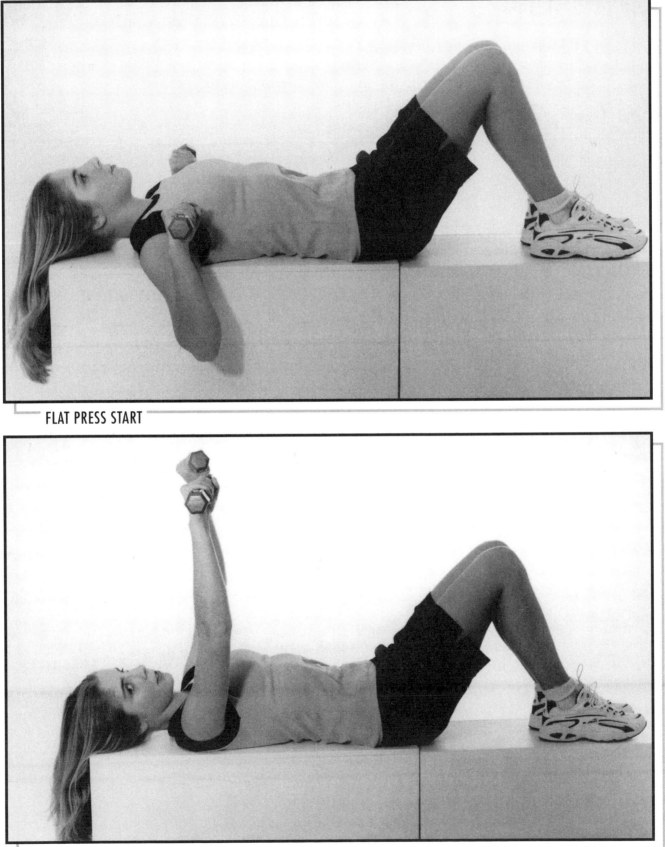

FLAT PRESS START

FLAT PRESS FINISH

2. DUMBBELL FLYE

This exercise develops, shapes, strengthens, and defines the entire chest/breast (pectoral) area, and helps add to the look of cleavage. There are fringe benefits for the upper arms, shoulders, and shoulder joints.

Stance: Holding a dumbbell in each hand, palms facing each other, lie on a flat exercise bench. Bend your knees and place the soles of your feet flat on the bench to prevent your back from arching. Extend your arms straight up, with your elbows very slightly bent. The dumbbells should be touching over the center of your chest.

Movement: With your elbows slightly bent, extend your arms outward and downward in an arclike movement until you feel a complete stretch in your chest muscles. Flexing your pectoral muscles as you go, return to the start position. Repeat the movement until you have completed your set. Without resting, move to your third chest exercise, the cross-bench pullover.

Tips: Beware the temptation to swing the dumbbells out and jerk them back in. Control them at all times. Don't lock your elbows. Keep them slightly bent throughout the movement—in the same position—as if they were slightly curved steel bars. Don't hold your breath. Breathe naturally.

Machines, Etc.: You may use the pec-dec machine in place of this exercise. You can do this exercise on an incline bench.

SETS, REPETITIONS, WEIGHTS (same as page 42, repeated here for review):

Set 1. Light: 12 reps flat press + 12 reps flat flye + 12 reps cross-bench pullover. Rest 15 seconds.

Set 2. Middle: 10 reps flat press + 10 reps flat flye + 10 reps cross-bench pullover. Rest 15 seconds.

Set 3. Heaviest: 8 reps flat press + 8 reps flat flye + 8 reps cross-bench pullover. Rest 15 seconds.

Reminder: See pages 36–37 for tips on heaviness of weights and raising weights.

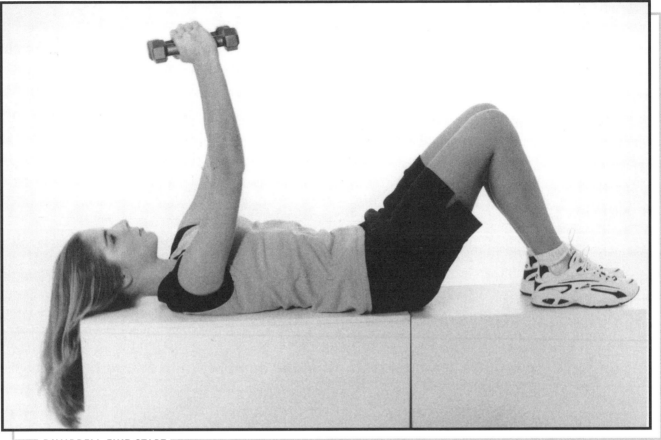

DUMBBELL FLYE START

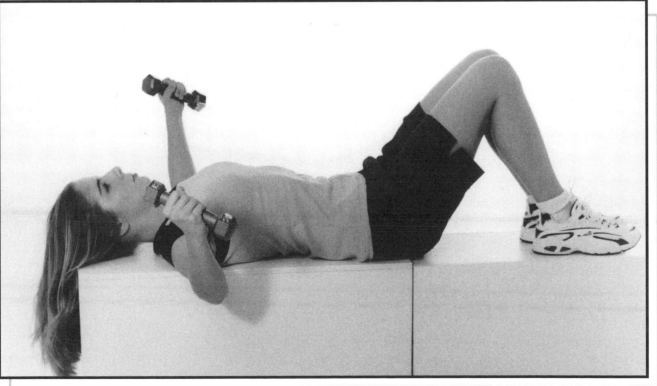

DUMBBELL FLYE FINISH

3. CROSS-BENCH PULLOVER

Develops, shapes, and firms the entire chest area. Also helps expand the rib cage and develop the back muscles.

Stance: Lie on a flat exercise bench with your knees bent and the soles of your feet flat on the bench to prevent your back from arching. Hold a dumbbell in your hands, palms upward, between your crossed thumbs. Extend your arms straight up so that the dumbbell is held directly over your forehead.

Movement: Extend the dumbbell behind you by lowering your arms and bending your elbows at the same time, until you cannot go any farther. Feel a full stretch in your chest muscles. Flex your chest muscles as you return to the start position, and give your muscles an extra-hard flex as you reach the start position. Repeat the movement until you have completed your set. Rest for fifteen seconds and do your next giant set of chest exercises.

Tips: Do not let the weight fall to the down position—maintain control at all times. Try to keep your back flat against the bench as you do the movements. Remember to breathe!

Machines, Etc.: You may perform this exercise with your feet on the ground and your shoulders resting at the edge of the bench.

SETS, REPETITIONS, WEIGHTS (same as page 42, repeated here for review):

Set 1. Light: 12 reps flat press + 12 reps flat flye + 12 reps cross-bench pullover. Rest 15 seconds.

Set 2. Middle: 10 reps flat press + 10 reps flat flye + 10 reps cross-bench pullover. Rest 15 seconds.

Set 3. Heaviest: 8 reps flat press + 8 reps flat flye + 8 reps cross-bench pullover. Rest 15 seconds.

Reminder: See pages 36–37 for tips on heaviness of weights and raising weights.

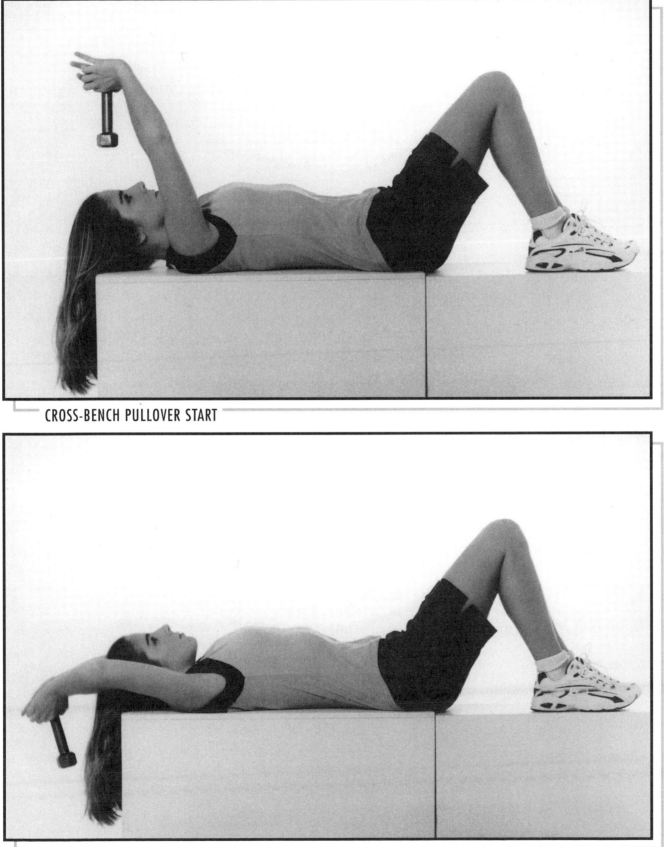

CROSS-BENCH PULLOVER START

CROSS-BENCH PULLOVER FINISH

SHOULDER ROUTINE

1. SIDE LATERAL

This exercise strengthens, develops, shapes, and defines the entire shoulder (deltoid) muscle, and helps strengthen the shoulder joints, shoulder blade, and collarbone. There are fringe benefits for the upper arms and wrists.

Stance: Stand with your feet a natural width apart. Hold a dumbbell in each hand with your arms extended down and your palms facing each other. The dumbbells should be almost touching each other at the center of your body.

Movement: Flexing your shoulder muscles as you go and making believe you're pouring a pitcher of water, extend your arms upward and outward until the dumbbells are shoulder height. In full control, return to the start position. Repeat the movement until you have completed your set. Without resting, move to your next shoulder exercise, the alternate front raise.

Tips: Don't rock back and forth as you work, and don't swing the dumbbells. Let your shoulders, not your back, do the work. Try not to extend the dumbbells higher than shoulder height.

Machines, Etc.: You may do this exercise on any side lateral machine.

SETS, REPETITIONS, WEIGHTS

Set 1. Light: 12 reps side lateral + 12 reps front lateral + 12 reps alternate shoulder press. Rest 15 seconds.

Set 2. Middle: 10 reps side lateral + 10 reps front lateral + 10 reps alternate shoulder press. Rest 15 seconds.

Set 3. Heaviest: 8 reps side lateral + 8 reps front lateral + 8 reps alternate shoulder press. Rest 15 seconds.

Reminder: See pages 36–37 for tips on heaviness of weights and raising weights.

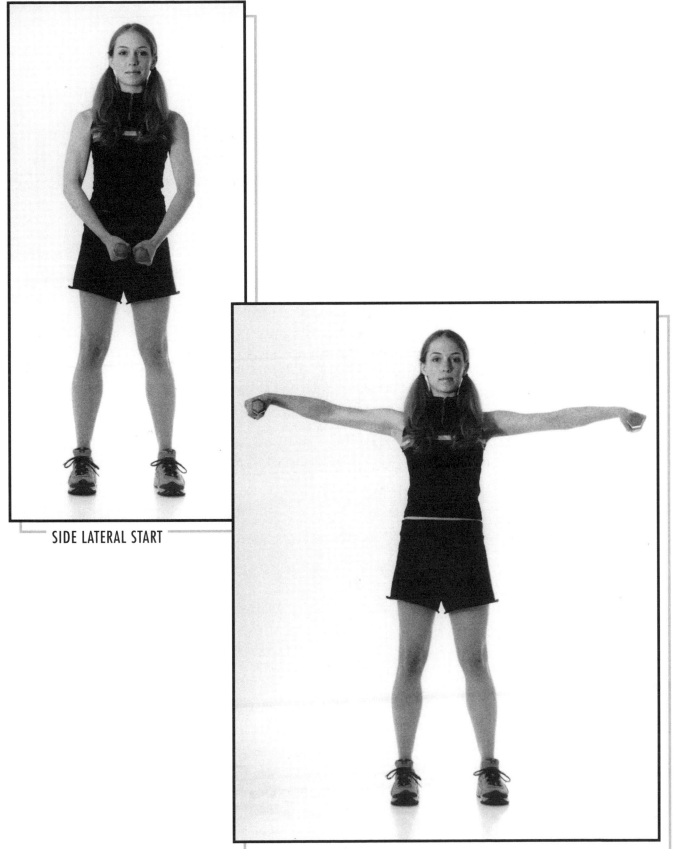

SIDE LATERAL START

SIDE LATERAL FINISH

2. ALTERNATE FRONT LATERAL

This exercise develops, shapes, strengthens, and defines the entire shoulder (deltoid) muscle, especially the front area, and helps strengthen the shoulder bones (scapula and clavicle). There are fringe benefits for the wrists and shoulder joints.

Stance: With your knees very slightly bent, stand with your feet shoulder width apart. Extend your arms straight down in front of you, holding a dumbbell in each hand, palms facing your body. (A dumbbell will be held in front of each thigh.)

Movement: With your elbows as straight as possible without locking them, and flexing your shoulder muscles as you go, extend one arm up until the dumbbell reaches shoulder height. Feeling the stretch in your shoulder muscle, return to the start position. Repeat for the other arm. Continue this alternate movement until you have completed your set. Without resting, move to your third shoulder exercise, the alternate shoulder press.

Tips: Don't swing the dumbbells to give yourself momentum. Keep your body steady—don't rock as you work. Lift the dumbbells only to shoulder height. Remember to breathe.

Machines, Etc.: You may use a barbell instead of dumbbells, and perform this exercise two arms at a time. You can also do this exercise two arms at a time with dumbbells.

SETS, REPETITIONS, WEIGHTS (same as page 48, repeated here for review):

Set 1. Light: 12 reps side lateral + 12 reps front lateral + 12 reps alternate shoulder press. Rest 15 seconds.

Set 2. Middle: 10 reps side lateral + 10 reps front lateral + 10 reps alternate shoulder press. Rest 15 seconds.

Set 3. Heaviest: 8 reps side lateral + 8 reps front lateral + 8 reps alternate shoulder press. Rest 15 seconds.

Reminder: See pages 36–37 for tips on heaviness of weights and raising weights.

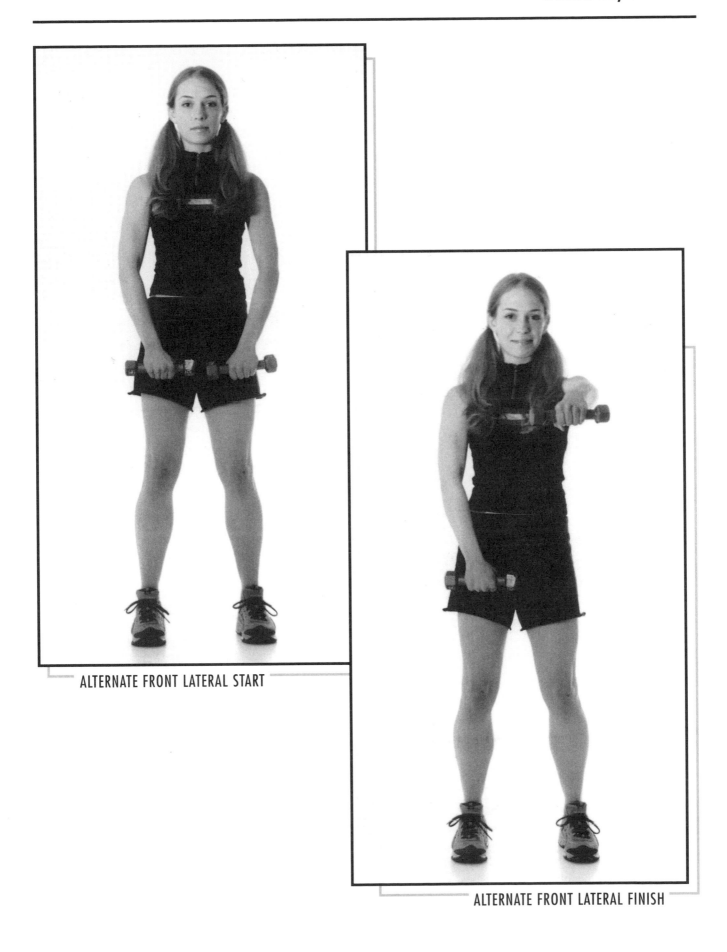

ALTERNATE FRONT LATERAL START

ALTERNATE FRONT LATERAL FINISH

3. ALTERNATE SHOULDER PRESS

This exercise strengthens, develops, shapes, and defines the entire shoulder (deltoid) muscle, and helps strengthen the shoulder blade (scapula) and collarbone (clavicle). There are fringe benefits for the trapezius and triceps muscles, and the wrists.

Stance: With a dumbbell held in each hand at shoulder height, palms facing away from your body, stand with your feet a natural width apart.

Movement: Flexing your shoulder muscles as you go, extend one arm upward until it's fully extended, but leave your elbow slightly bent. Return to the start position. Repeat the movement for the other arm. Repeat this alternative movement until you have completed your set. Rest for 15 seconds and do your next giant set of shoulder exercises.

Tips: Maintain full control as you raise and lower the dumbbells. Don't lock your elbows on the up movement. Do complete movements—all the way up, all the way down. Don't allow yourself to rock back and forth—keep your body steady. Let your shoulders, not your back, do the work.

Machines, Etc.: You can do this exercise on any shoulder press machine. You can also do this seated, or with two arms at a time standing or seated.

SETS, REPETITIONS, WEIGHTS (same as page 48, repeated here for review):

Set 1. Light: 12 reps side lateral + 12 reps front lateral + 12 reps alternate shoulder press. Rest 15 seconds.

Set 2. Middle: 10 reps side lateral + 10 reps front lateral + 10 reps alternate shoulder press. Rest 15 seconds.

Set 3. Heaviest: 8 reps side lateral + 8 reps front lateral + 8 reps alternate shoulder press. Rest 15 seconds.

Reminder: See pages 36–37 for tips on heaviness of weights and raising weights.

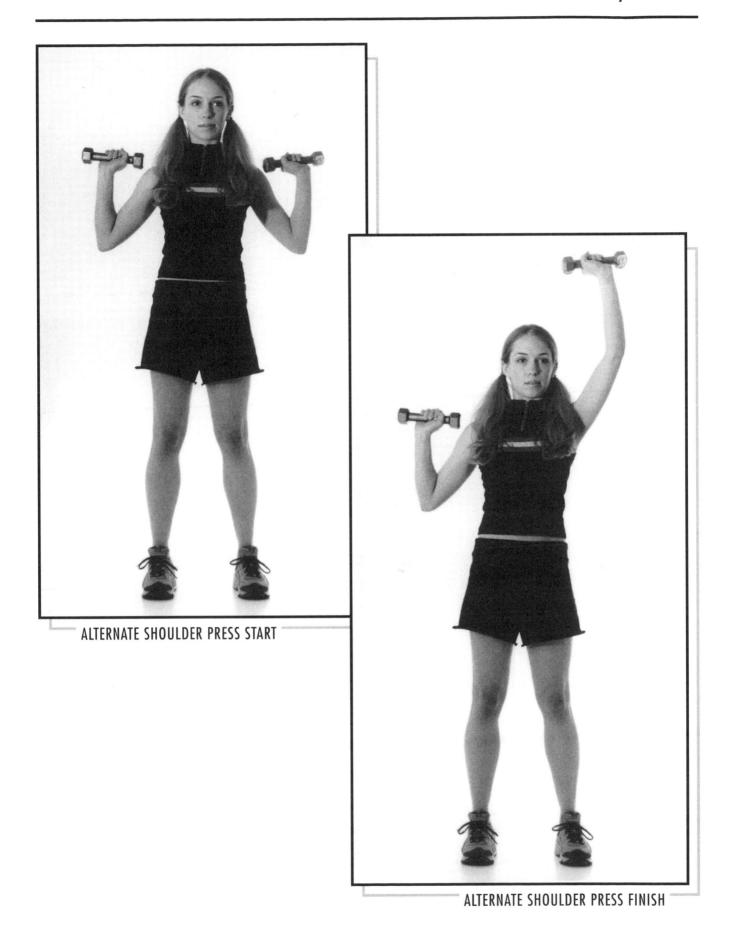

ALTERNATE SHOULDER PRESS START

ALTERNATE SHOULDER PRESS FINISH

BICEPS ROUTINE

1. SIMULTANEOUS CURL

This exercise develops, shapes, and defines the entire biceps muscle, and strengthens the underlying bone (humerus), along with the wrist bones. There are fringe benefits for the forearm.

Stance:
Stand with your feet a natural width apart, holding a dumbbell in each hand, palms facing your body. Your arms should be straight down at your sides and close to your body.

Movement:
Flexing your biceps muscles as you go, with your wrists very slightly curled toward the front of your body and bending at the elbows, curl your arms upward toward your shoulders, until the dumbbells are nearly touching your upper chest area. Without resting, return to the start position. Repeat the movement until you have completed your set. Without resting, move to your next biceps exercise, the alternate hammer curl.

Tips:
Don't rock back and forth as you move the dumbbells.

Machines, Etc.:
You may perform this exercise on any biceps curl machine. You can also do this by alternating one arm at a time.

SETS, REPETITIONS, WEIGHTS

Set 1. Light: 12 reps simultaneous curl + 12 reps alternate hammer curl + 12 reps concentration curl. Rest 15 seconds.

Set 2. Middle: 10 reps simultaneous curl + 10 reps alternate hammer curl + 10 reps concentration curl. Rest 15 seconds.

Set 3. Heaviest: 8 reps simultaneous curl + 8 reps alternate hammer curl + 8 reps concentration curl. Rest 15 seconds.

Reminder:
See pages 36–37 for tips on heaviness of weights and raising weights.

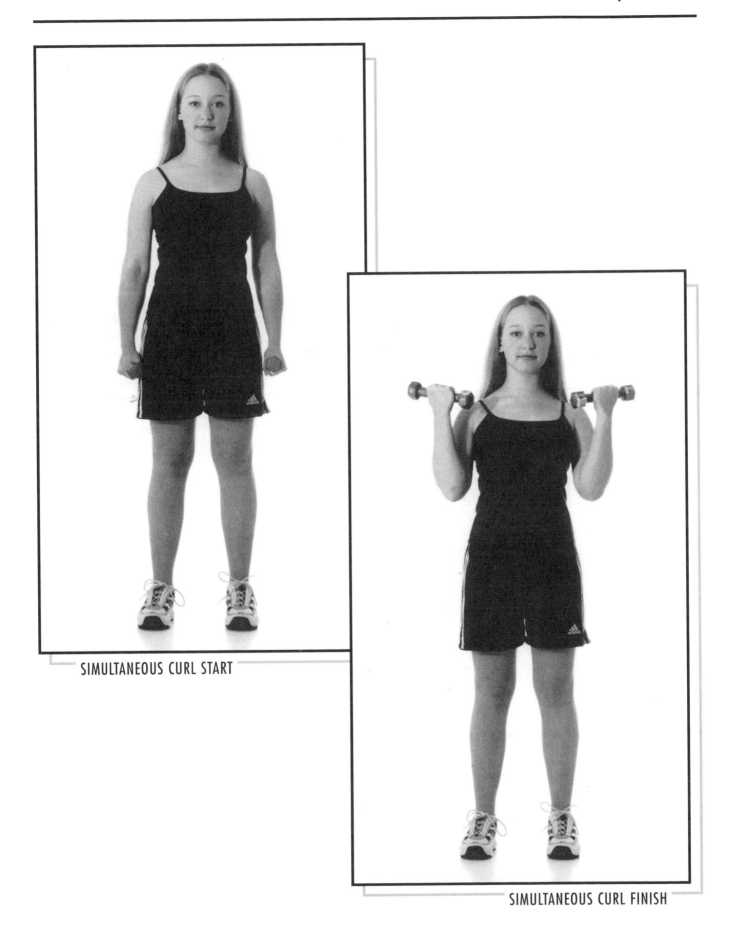

SIMULTANEOUS CURL START

SIMULTANEOUS CURL FINISH

2. ALTERNATE HAMMER CURL

This exercise develops and shapes the entire biceps muscle and strengthens the forearm.

Stance: Stand with your feet a natural width apart. Hold a dumbbell in each hand, palms facing your body. Let your arms hang down at the sides of your body.

Movement: With palms facing your body and the dumbbells in the "hammer" position (see the start photo), curl one arm up to your shoulder as far as you can go. Flex your biceps muscle and return to the start position. Without stopping, immediately repeat the movement for the other arm. Continue this alternating curling movement until you have completed your set. Without resting, move to your third biceps exercise, the concentration curl.

Tips: Don't rock your body; stay steady. Remember to flex your biceps muscles on the upward movement and feel the stretch on the downward movement.

Machines, Etc.: You may perform this exercise two arms at a time, standing, seated, or lying on a flat or incline bench. You can substitute a biceps machine exercise for this exercise.

SETS, REPETITIONS, WEIGHTS (same as page 54, repeated here for review)

Set 1. Light: 12 reps simultaneous curl + 12 reps alternate hammer curl + 12 reps concentration curl. Rest 15 seconds.
Set 2. Middle: 10 reps simultaneous curl + 10 reps alternate hammer curl + 10 reps concentration curl. Rest 15 seconds.
Set 3. Heaviest: 8 reps simultaneous curl + 8 reps alternate hammer curl + 8 reps concentration curl. Rest 15 seconds.

Reminder: See pages 36–37 for tips on heaviness of weights and raising weights.

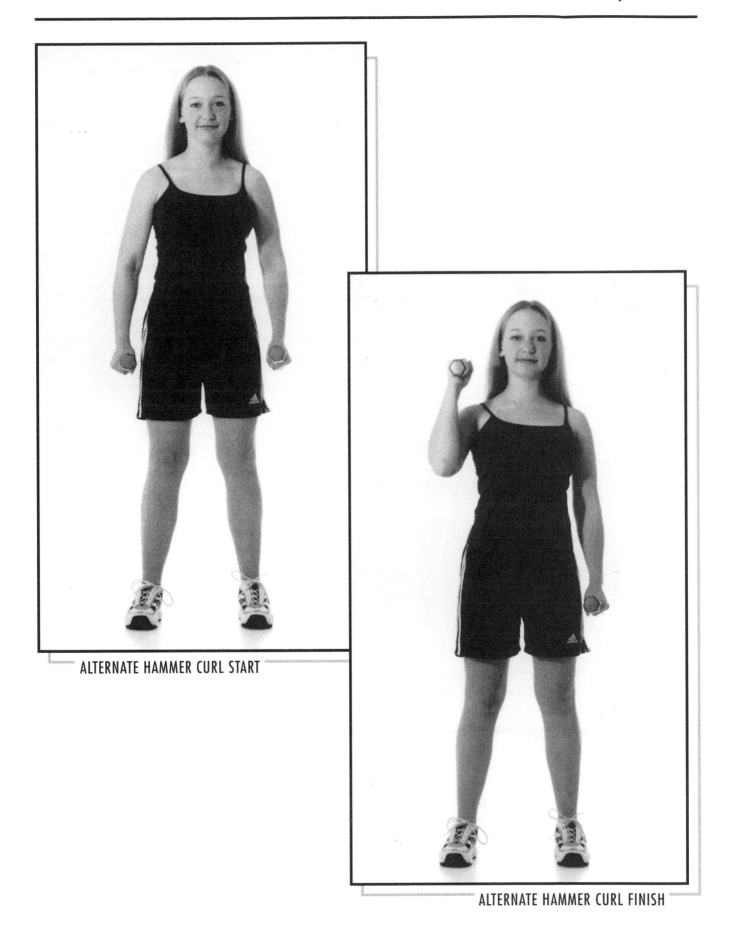

ALTERNATE HAMMER CURL START

ALTERNATE HAMMER CURL FINISH

3. CONCENTRATION CURL

This exercise strengthens, develops, shapes, and defines the entire biceps muscle, and strengthens the underlying bone (humerus). There are fringe benefits for the wrist, forearm, and triceps muscles and bones.

Stance: Holding a dumbbell in your right hand, palm away from your body, and wrist curled slightly upward, bend over with your legs about ten inches wider than shoulder width apart. Place your right elbow on your inner thigh about six inches above the knee. Extend your arm downward for the start position.

Movement: Flexing your biceps muscle as you go, curl your working arm upward toward your face as far as you can go (approximately chin height). Give your biceps muscle an extra flex and return to the start position, feeling the stretch in your biceps. Repeat the movement until you have completed your set. Repeat the set for your other arm. Rest for fifteen seconds and do your next giant set of biceps exercises.

Tips: Try to keep your head down throughout the movement. Make believe you are going to punch yourself in the face with the dumbbell each time. Don't swing the dumbbell up and down. Keep your wrist slightly curled throughout the movement. Maintain control at all times. Don't hold your breath. Breathe naturally.

Machines, Etc.: You can do this exercise using a "preacher bench." It's called the preacher curl.

SETS, REPETITIONS, WEIGHTS (same as page 54, repeated here for review)

Set 1. Light: 12 reps simultaneous curl + 12 reps alternate hammer curl + 12 reps concentration curl. Rest 15 seconds.

Set 2. Middle: 10 reps simultaneous curl + 10 reps alternate hammer curl + 10 reps concentration curl. Rest 15 seconds.

Set 3. Heaviest: 8 reps simultaneous curl + 8 reps alternate hammer curl + 8 reps concentration curl. Rest 15 seconds.

Reminder: See pages 36–37 for tips on heaviness of weights and raising weights.

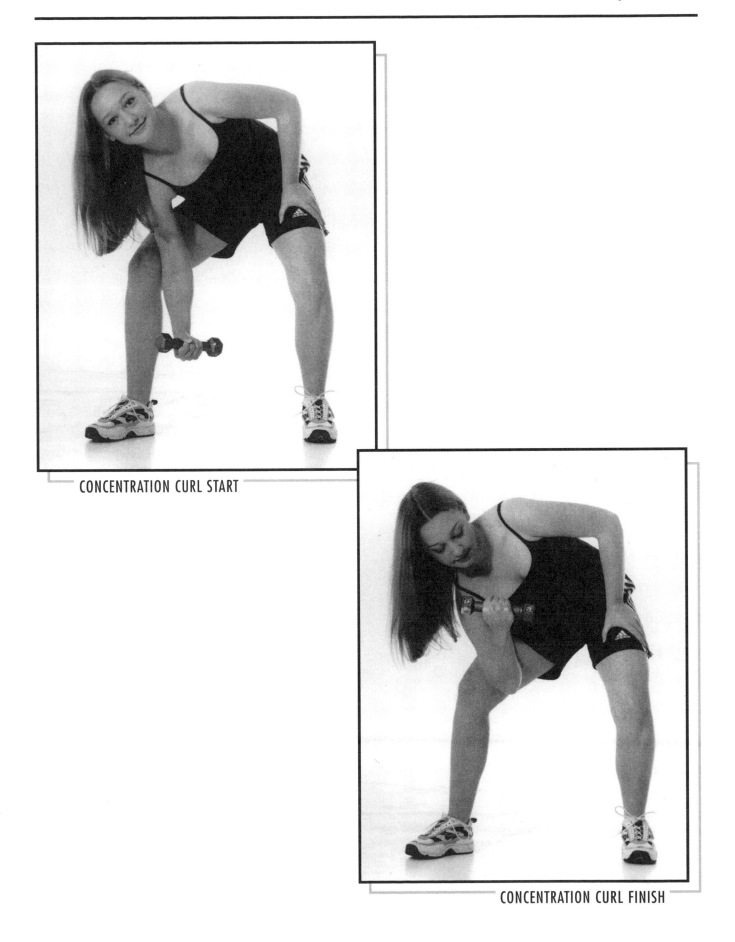

CONCENTRATION CURL START

CONCENTRATION CURL FINISH

TRICEPS ROUTINE

1. DOUBLE-ARM KICKBACK

This exercise develops, shapes, strengthens, and defines the entire triceps muscle and strengthens the underlying bone (the humerus). There are fringe benefits for the wrist, elbow, and shoulder joints.

Stance: Stand with one foot about seven inches in front of the other, and, bending at the waist and knees, hold a dumbbell in each hand, palms facing your body. Bend your arms at the elbows so that the dumbbells are about upper chest height. Your elbows should be close to your body, nearly touching your waist.

Movement: Keeping your arms close to your body, and flexing your triceps as you go, extend your arms back as far as possible. Give your triceps muscles an extra flex. Without resting, return to the start position and feel the stretch in your triceps. Repeat the movement until you have completed your set. Without resting, move to your next triceps exercise, the one-arm overhead.

Tips: Keep your arms close to your body throughout the exercise. Don't jerk the dumbbells back; control your movements. Don't hold your breath. Breathe naturally.

Machines, Etc.: You may perform this exercise with a curved triceps pull-down bar, using any machine pulley device.

SETS, REPETITIONS, WEIGHTS

Set 1. Light: 12 reps double-arm kickback + 12 reps one-arm overhead + 12 reps close bench press. Rest 15 seconds.
Set 2. Middle: 10 reps double-arm kickback + 10 reps one-arm overhead + 10 reps close bench press. Rest 15 seconds.
Set 3. Heaviest: 8 reps double-arm kickback + 8 reps one-arm overhead + 8 reps close bench press. Rest 15 seconds.

Reminder: See pages 36–37 for tips on heaviness of weights and raising weights.

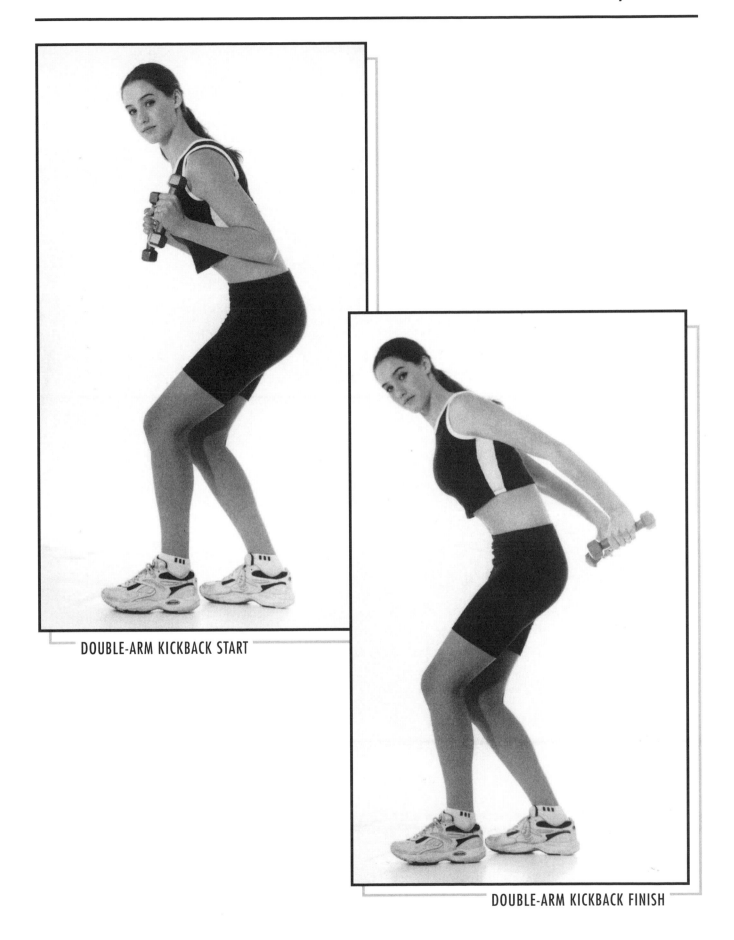

DOUBLE-ARM KICKBACK START

DOUBLE-ARM KICKBACK FINISH

2. ONE-ARM OVERHEAD

This exercise strengthens, develops, shapes, and defines the entire triceps muscle, and strengthens the underlying bone (humerus). There are fringe benefits for the elbows and wrists.

Stance:

Sit on a flat exercise bench or a chair, holding a dumbbell in your right hand, palm facing the side of your body, and your arm extended fully upward. Let your biceps muscle nearly touch your ear. Place your left hand on your right thigh or on your right upper arm to feel your triceps muscle working. This serves a double purpose of supporting your arm and feeling your triceps muscle work as you go.

Movement:

In full control, and feeling the stretch in your triceps muscle as you go, lower the dumbbell behind your head by unbending your elbow and allowing the dumbbell to descend until you cannot go any farther, all the time keeping your upper arm close to your ear. Without resting, and flexing your triceps muscle as you go, return to the start position. Give your triceps muscle an extra flex, and repeat the movement until you have completed your set. Without resting, move to your next triceps exercise, the close bench press.

Tips:

If your elbow seems extra weak, brace it with your nonworking hand (instead of placing it on your triceps).

Machines, Etc:

You may perform this exercise using any triceps extension machine.

SETS, REPETITIONS, WEIGHTS (same as page 60, repeated here for review):

Set 1. Light: 12 reps double-arm kickback + 12 reps one-arm overhead + 12 reps close bench press. Rest 15 seconds.

Set 2. Middle: 10 reps double-arm kickback + 10 reps one-arm overhead + 10 reps close bench press. Rest 15 seconds.

Set 3. Heaviest: 8 reps double-arm kickback + 8 reps one-arm overhead + 8 reps close bench press. Rest 15 seconds.

Reminder:

See pages 36–37 for tips on heaviness of weights and raising weights.

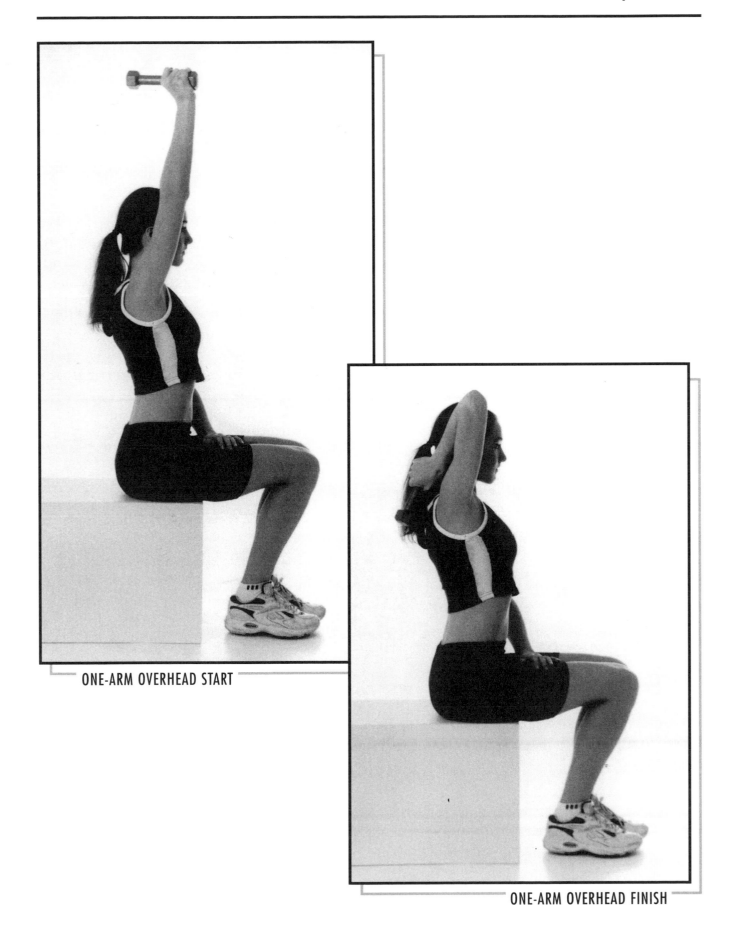

ONE-ARM OVERHEAD START

ONE-ARM OVERHEAD FINISH

3. CLOSE BENCH PRESS

This exercise develops, shapes, strengthens, and defines the entire triceps muscle.

Stance: Lie on a flat exercise bench with your knees bent and the soles of your feet flat on the bench so you don't arch your back. Grip a dumbbell with both hands, palms facing upward. Hold the dumbbell close to the center of your chest.

Movement: Flexing your triceps muscles as you go, raise your arms upward until they are fully extended. Give your triceps muscles an extra-hard flex and, keeping your elbows close to your body, return to the start position. Feel the stretch in your triceps and repeat the movement until you have completed your set. Rest for fifteen seconds and do the next giant set of your triceps exercises.

Tips: To make sure that your triceps do the work, be sure to keep your upper arms close to your body throughout the exercise.

Machines, Etc.: You may use a regular barbell for this exercise.

SETS, REPETITIONS, WEIGHTS (same as page 60, repeated here for review):

Set 1. Light: 12 reps double-arm kickback + 12 reps one-arm overhead + 12 reps close bench press. Rest 15 seconds.

Set 2. Middle: 10 reps double-arm kickback + 10 reps one-arm overhead + 10 reps close bench press. Rest 15 seconds.

Set 3. Heaviest: 8 reps double-arm kickback + 8 reps one-arm overhead + 8 reps close bench press. Rest 15 seconds.

Reminder: See pages 36–37 for tips on heaviness of weights and raising weights.

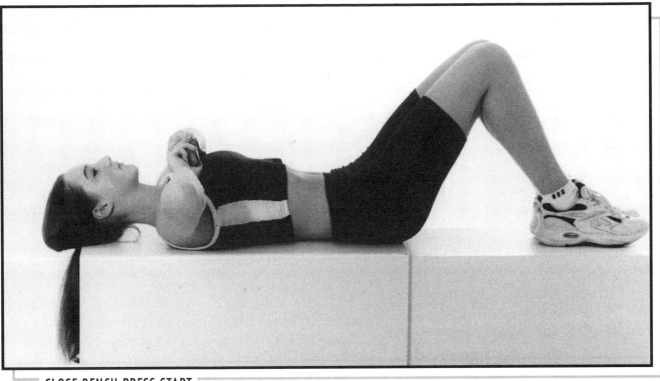

CLOSE BENCH PRESS START

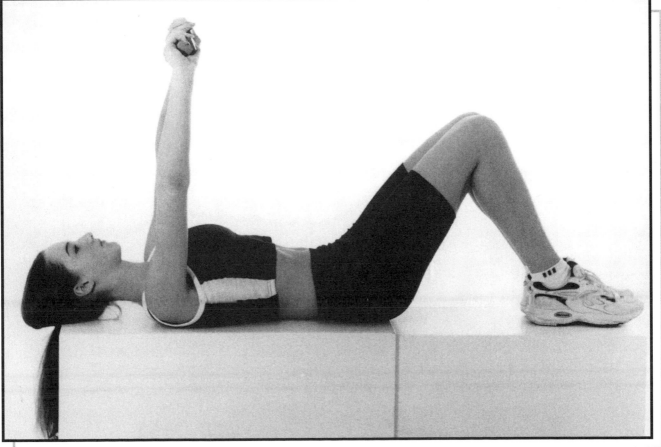

CLOSE BENCH PRESS FINISH

BACK ROUTINE

1. BENT LATERAL

This exercise develops, shapes, strengthens, and defines the rear and side shoulder (deltoid) muscles, and strengthens the back and shoulder muscles in general. It also strengthens the spinal column.

Stance: Stand with your feet a natural width apart, holding a dumbbell in each hand, with your palms facing each other. Bend over until your upper body is nearly parallel to the floor and extend your arms straight down in front of you in the center of your body. The dumbbells should be nearly touching each other at about knee height.

Movement: Keeping your wrists slightly bent, and flexing your side and rear shoulder muscles as you go, extend your arms outward until your arms are almost parallel to the floor. Willfully flex your shoulder muscles and return to the start position. Feel the stretch in your shoulder muscles. Repeat the movement until you have completed your set. Without resting, move to your next back exercise, the seated lateral.

Tips: Keep your upper body (torso) parallel to the floor throughout the movement. Don't jerk the dumbbells. Use control. This is not an easy exercise to do; you'll get used to it.

Machines, Etc.: You may perform this exercise using any spaced-apart floor pulley machine. Set the weights at ten pounds.

SETS, REPETITIONS, WEIGHTS

Set 1. Light: 12 reps bent lateral + 12 reps seated lateral + 12 reps double-arm upright row. Rest 15 seconds.

Set 2. Middle: 10 reps bent lateral + 10 reps seated lateral + 10 reps double-arm upright row. Rest 15 seconds.

Set 3. Heaviest: 8 reps bent lateral + 8 reps seated lateral + 8 reps double-arm upright row. Rest 15 seconds.

Reminder: See pages 36–37 for tips on heaviness of weights and raising weights.

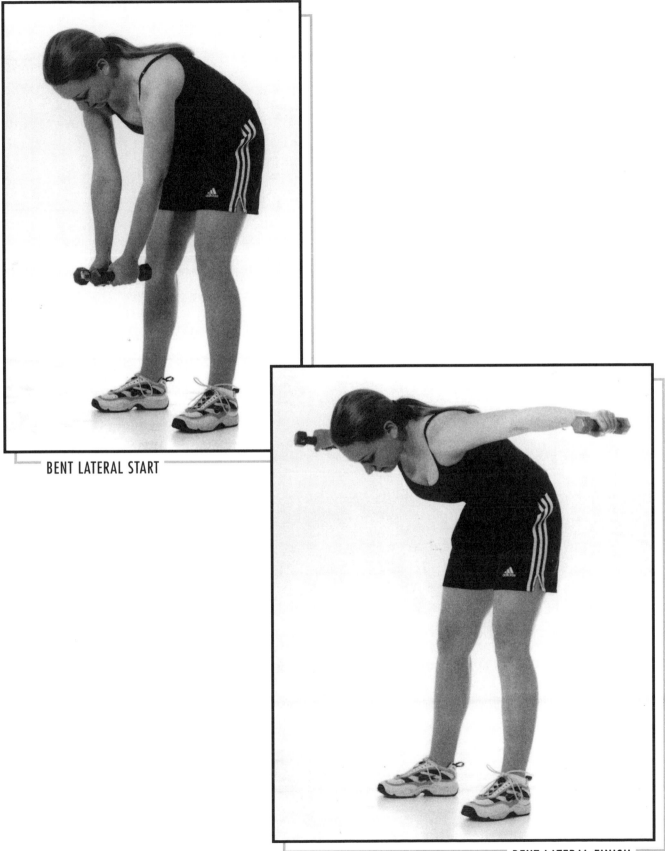

BENT LATERAL START

BENT LATERAL FINISH

2. SEATED LATERAL

This exercise develops, shapes, strengthens, and defines the upper back and trapezius muscles and strengthens the upper back muscles in general.

Stance: Holding a dumbbell in each hand, sit at the edge of a flat exercise bench or chair and lean forward until your chest is a few inches away from your thighs. Palms facing to the rear, hold the dumbbells behind your legs, letting the ends of the dumbbells touch.

Movement: Flexing your upper back muscles as you go, and keeping the dumbbells close to your body, raise the dumbbells up and back, rotating them ninety degrees as you go so that when you reach hip level, the dumbbells are angled to the front and your palms are facing front. Willfully flex your upper back muscles by making believe you're trying to squeeze a pencil in the middle of your back. Return to the start position and feel the stretch in your upper back. Repeat the movement until you have completed your set. Without resting, move to your third back exercise, the double-arm upright row.

Tips: Keep your arms close to your sides throughout the exercise.

Machines, Etc.: You can substitute a T-bar rowing machine for this exercise. Use a five-pound plate, or set the weight at ten pounds.

SETS, REPETITIONS, WEIGHTS (same as page 66, repeated here for review):

Set 1. Light: 12 reps bent lateral + 12 reps seated lateral + 12 reps double-arm upright row. Rest 15 seconds.

Set 2. Middle: 10 reps bent lateral + 10 reps seated lateral + 10 reps double-arm upright row. Rest 15 seconds.

Set 3. Heaviest: 8 reps bent lateral + 8 reps seated lateral + 8 reps double-arm upright row. Rest 15 seconds.

Reminder: See pages 36–37 for tips on heaviness of weights and raising weights.

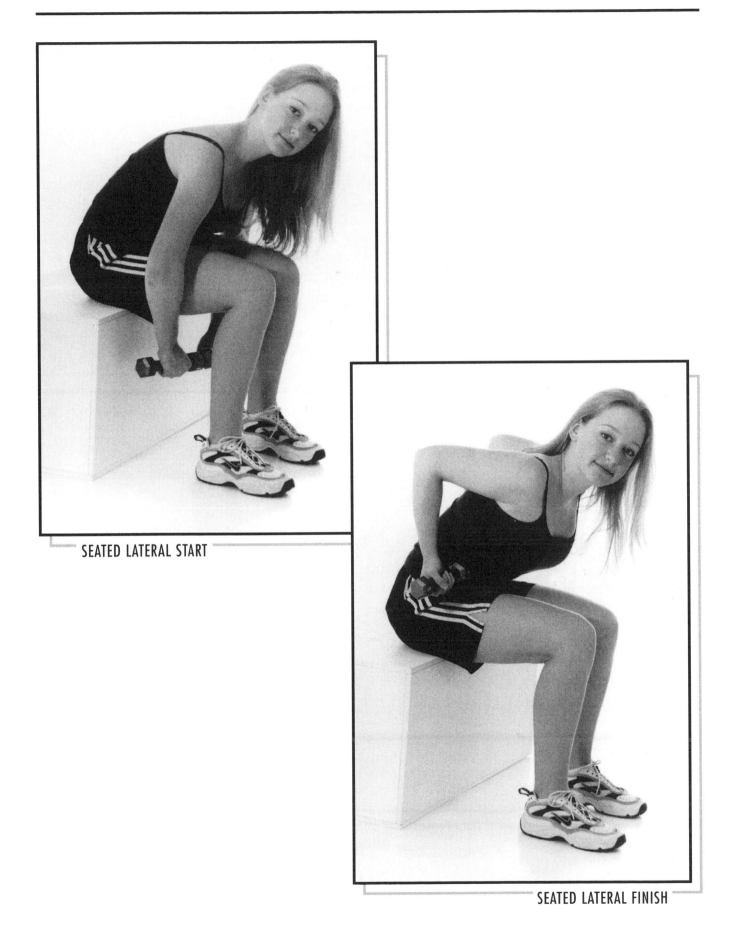

SEATED LATERAL START

SEATED LATERAL FINISH

3. DOUBLE-ARM UPRIGHT ROW

This exercise develops, shapes, strengthens, and defines the entire trapezius muscle, and strengthens and builds the bones in the entire spinal column. It also helps strengthen the shoulder joints. There are fringe benefits for the biceps.

Stance: Holding a dumbbell in each hand, palms facing your body, stand with your feet a natural width apart. Extend your arms fully downward, positioning each dumbbell in the center of a thigh.

Movement: Flexing your trapezius muscles as you go, extending your elbows outward and keeping the dumbbells close to your body, raise the dumbbells until they reach nearly chin height. In full control, return to the start position. Feel the stretch in your trapezius, shoulder, and upper back muscles. Repeat the movement until you have completed your set. Rest for fifteen seconds and do the next giant set of your back exercises.

Tips: Keep the dumbbells close to your body as you move. On the final up position, your elbows should be approximately shoulder height, and parallel to the floor. Don't cheat the movement: Go all the way up and all the way down in full control. Don't hold your breath. Breathe naturally.

Machines, Etc: You may do this exercise on any floor pulley machine.

SETS, REPETITIONS, WEIGHTS (same as page 66, repeated here for review):

Set 1. Light: 12 reps bent lateral + 12 reps seated lateral + 12 reps double-arm upright row. Rest 15 seconds.

Set 2. Middle: 10 reps bent lateral + 10 reps seated lateral + 10 reps double-arm upright row. Rest 15 seconds.

Set 3. Heaviest: 8 reps bent lateral + 8 reps seated lateral + 8 reps double-arm upright row. Rest 15 seconds.

Reminder: See pages 36–37 for tips on heaviness of weights and raising weights.

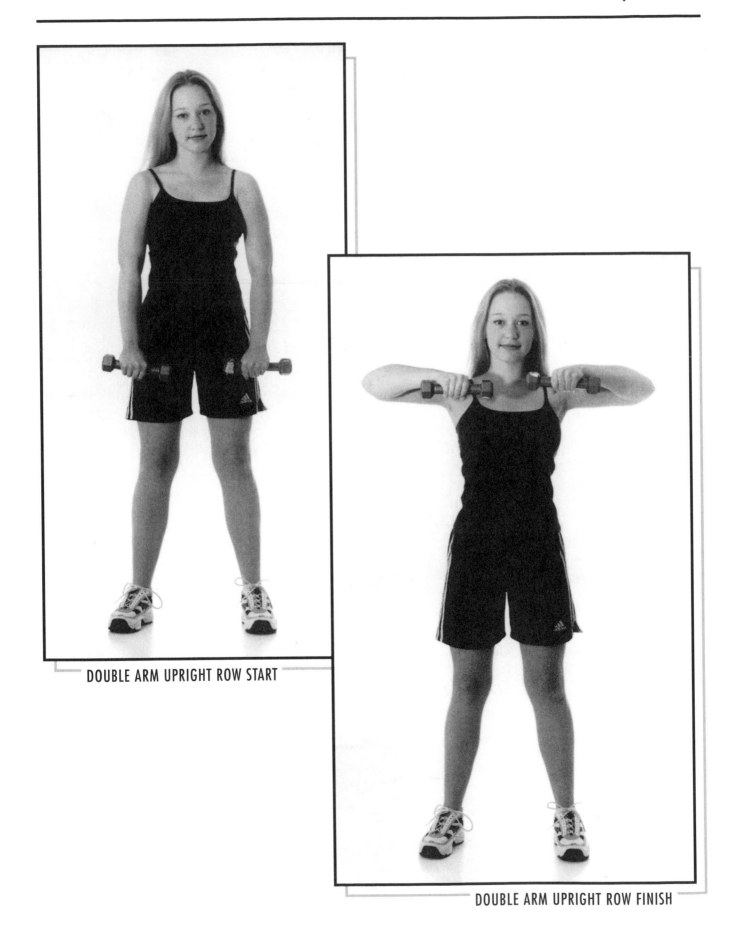

DOUBLE ARM UPRIGHT ROW START

DOUBLE ARM UPRIGHT ROW FINISH

REVIEW OF EXERCISES FOUND IN THIS CHAPTER

Chest

Flat press
Dumbbell flye
Cross-bench pullover
    Extra: Incline press
           Incline flye

Shoulders

Side lateral
Alternate front lateral
Alternate shoulder press
    Extra: Simultaneous front lateral
           Simultaneous shoulder press

Biceps

Simultaneous curl
Alternate hammer curl
Concentration curl
    Extra: Alternate curl
           Simultaneous hammer

Triceps

Double-arm kickback
One-arm overhead
Close bench press
    Extra: One-arm kickback
           Double-arm overhead

Back

Bent lateral
Seated lateral
Double-arm upright row
    Extra: Seated bent lateral
           One-arm upright row

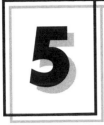

5 WORKOUT DAY TWO:

LOWER BODY

Now it's time to do your day two workout. Here you will exercise your lower body: thighs, hips/buttocks, abdominals, and calves. As before, you'll be doing this workout every other time you work out. Unlike workout day one, you will be required here to do five exercises for each body part—except for calves, which require only three.

Why the extra work? As mentioned before, most women need extra work on the thighs, hips/buttocks, and abdomen to burn maximum fat and get ultimate definition and shaping in the minimum amount of time. You will be working in giant sets.

You'll do your thighs first because they're strong and will welcome the wake-up call to start your workout. Next you will turn to your hip/butt area, because that area is closely related to your thighs, and will be made ready and alert by the thigh workout. Then come your abdominals, which require a good deal of effort but are totally unrelated to your thighs or hips/buttocks, so you'll be able to exercise them without exhaustion. Finally, to have something to look forward to, you'll do the easy calf exercises last.

Before you start this workout day, you may want to review the section on how to do the day two workout in chapter 3. Then simply follow the photographs and exercise instructions. In time, you may not even need the instructions anymore.

THIGH ROUTINE

1. Plié Squat

This exercise develops, shapes, tones, and defines the entire front thigh muscles. There are fringe benefits for the hip/buttock area. In addition, the hip joints, thighbones, and spinal column are strengthened.

Stance: Holding a dumbbell with both hands at the center of your body with palms facing your body, stand with your feet about ten inches wider than shoulder width apart and point your toes outward. Extend your arms down and keep your elbows slightly bent. Keep your back straight and look straight ahead.

Movement: Feeling the stretch in your front thigh muscles as you go, descend to an approximate forty-five-degree bend in your knees. Flexing your front thigh muscles as you go, return to the start position. Give your quadriceps an extra-hard flex, and repeat the movement until you have completed your set. Without resting, move to the next exercise in this routine, the lunge.

Tips: Keep your heels flat to the ground as you work. You may have to take a wide stance in order to do that. Keep your eyes straight ahead and your back straight as you descend and ascend.

Machines, Etc.: You may also do this exercise at any squat machine.

SETS, REPETITIONS, WEIGHTS

Set 1. Light: 12 reps squat + 12 reps lunge + 12 reps leg curl + 12 reps front squat + 12 reps hack squat. Rest 15 seconds.

Set 2. Middle: 10 reps squat + 10 reps lunge + 10 reps leg curl + 10 reps front squat + 10 reps hack squat. Rest 15 seconds.

Set 3. Heaviest: 8 reps squat + 8 reps lunge + 8 reps leg curl + 8 reps front squat + 8 reps hack squat. Rest 15 seconds.

Reminder: See pages 36–37 for tips on heaviness of weights and raising weights.

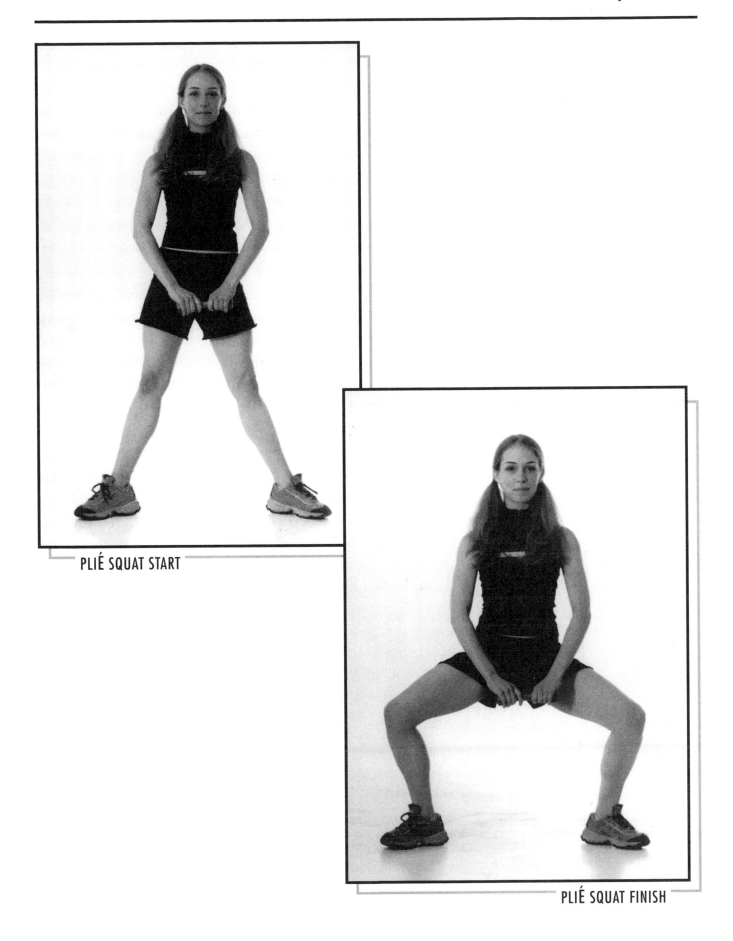

PLIÉ SQUAT START

PLIÉ SQUAT FINISH

2. Lunge

This exercise develops, shapes, tones, and defines the entire front thigh area; helps lift and shape the buttocks; and helps tighten and tone the hip/buttock area. In addition, the thigh, knee, and anklebones are strengthened.

Stance: Stand with your feet in a natural position, keeping your back straight and looking straight ahead. Hold a dumbbell in each hand, palms facing your body, with your arms straight down at your sides.

Movement: Keeping your knee aligned with your toe, bending at the knee, step forward with one foot (about two feet) until you can just about see your toes. (If you can't see your toes, you've stepped too far.) Feel the flex in your stepping front thigh muscle and the stretch in your nonstepping front thigh muscle. In full control, return to the start position and give both thighs an extra-hard flex. Repeat the movement for the other leg. Continue this alternate lunging movement until you have completed your set. Without resting, move to your next thigh exercise, the leg curl.

Tips: At first you may stumble and feel awkward. Don't worry. In time you will do this with no problem. Don't bounce as you lunge forward and back. Make sure your working knee is not extended beyond your toes.

Machines, Etc.: You may do leg presses on any leg press machine in place of this exercise.

SETS, REPETITIONS, WEIGHTS (same as page 74, repeated here for review):

Set 1. Light: 12 reps squat + 12 reps lunge + 12 reps leg curl + 12 reps front squat + 12 reps hack squat. Rest 15 seconds.

Set 2. Middle: 10 reps squat + 10 reps lunge + 10 reps leg curl + 10 reps front squat + 10 reps hack squat. Rest 15 seconds.

Set 3. Heaviest: 8 reps squat + 8 reps lunge + 8 reps leg curl + 8 reps front squat + 8 reps hack squat. Rest 15 seconds.

Reminder: See pages 36–37 for tips on heaviness of weights and raising weights.

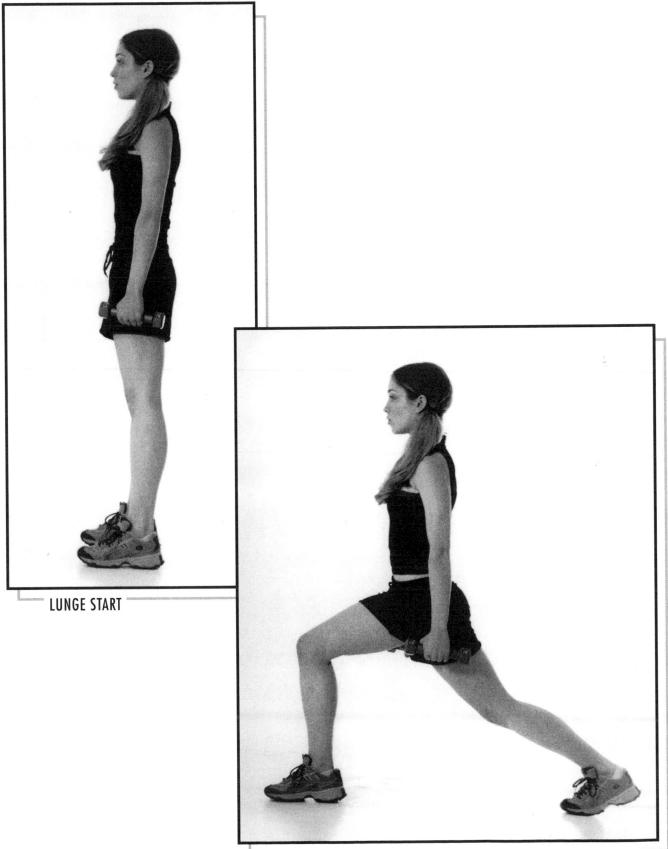

LUNGE START

LUNGE FINISH

3. Leg Curl

This exercise tightens, tones, shapes, and defines the back thigh muscles, and helps strengthen the knee and shinbones. '

Stance:

With a dumbbell placed between your feet, lie facedown on the floor or a flat exercise bench. Extend your legs straight out behind you with your arms crossed in front of you.

Movement:

Bending your knees and keeping the pressure on your back thigh muscles as you go, raise your lower legs until they are nearly perpendicular to the floor. Flexing your back thigh muscles as hard as possible, return to the start position. Repeat the movement until you have completed your set. Without resting, move to the next thigh exercise, the front squat.

Tips:

If you squeeze your ankles together, you'll be better able to keep the pressure on your back thigh muscles. Don't do this exercise without sneakers, and especially not barefoot. You'll hurt your feet—and the dumbbell may slip! Don't swing the dumbbell up and down. Maintain control throughout the movement.

Machines, Etc.:

You may perform this exercise on any leg curl machine.

SETS, REPETITIONS, WEIGHTS (same as page 74, repeated here for review):

Set 1. Light: 12 reps squat + 12 reps lunge + 12 reps leg curl + 12 reps front squat + 12 reps hack squat. Rest 15 seconds.

Set 2. Middle: 10 reps squat + 10 reps lunge + 10 reps leg curl + 10 reps front squat + 10 reps hack squat. Rest 15 seconds.

Set 3. Heaviest: 8 reps squat + 8 reps lunge + 8 reps leg curl + 8 reps front squat + 8 reps hack squat. Rest 15 seconds.

Reminder:

See pages 36–37 for tips on heaviness of weights and raising weights.

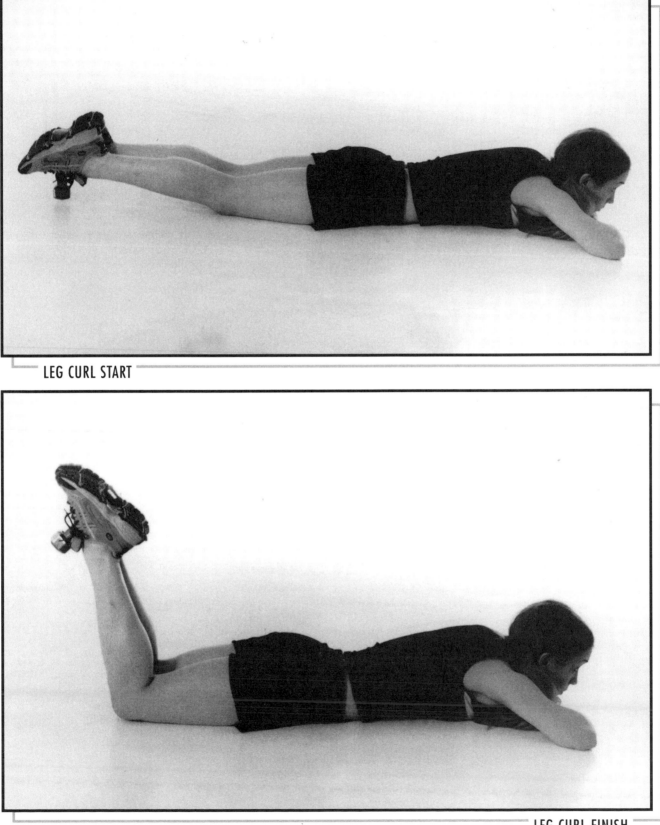

LEG CURL START

LEG CURL FINISH

4. Front Squat

Develops, shapes, tones, and defines the front thigh muscles. Helps tighten and tone the hip/buttock area, and in addition strengthens the hip joints, thighbones, and spinal column.

Stance:
Stand with your feet a natural width apart and your toes angled out. Hold a dumbbell in each hand, and cross your arms above your chest. The ends of the dumbbells should be touching your shoulders. Look straight ahead and keep your back straight.

Movement:
Keeping your upper body straight, feel the stretch in your front thighs as you descend to a squat position (descend until your thighs are slightly higher than parallel to the floor). Flex your front thighs as you return to the start position. Give your front thighs an extra-hard flex. Repeat the movement until you have completed your set. Without resting, move to your final thigh exercise, the hack squat.

Tips:
Sink to the ground on the down movement, and lead with your chest and chin on the up movement. Keep your eyes straight ahead and your back straight as you work.

Machines, Etc.:
You may balance a barbell on your chest instead of using the dumbbells. You can also substitute the leg press done on any leg press machine for this or any other squat.

SETS, REPETITIONS, WEIGHTS (same as page 74, repeated here for review):

Set 1. Light: 12 reps squat + 12 reps lunge + 12 reps leg curl + 12 reps front squat + 12 reps hack squat. Rest 15 seconds.

Set 2. Middle: 10 reps squat + 10 reps lunge + 10 reps leg curl + 10 reps front squat + 10 reps hack squat. Rest 15 seconds.

Set 3. Heaviest: 8 reps squat + 8 reps lunge + 8 reps leg curl + 8 reps front squat + 8 reps hack squat. Rest 15 seconds.

Reminder:
See pages 36–37 for tips on heaviness of weights and raising weights.

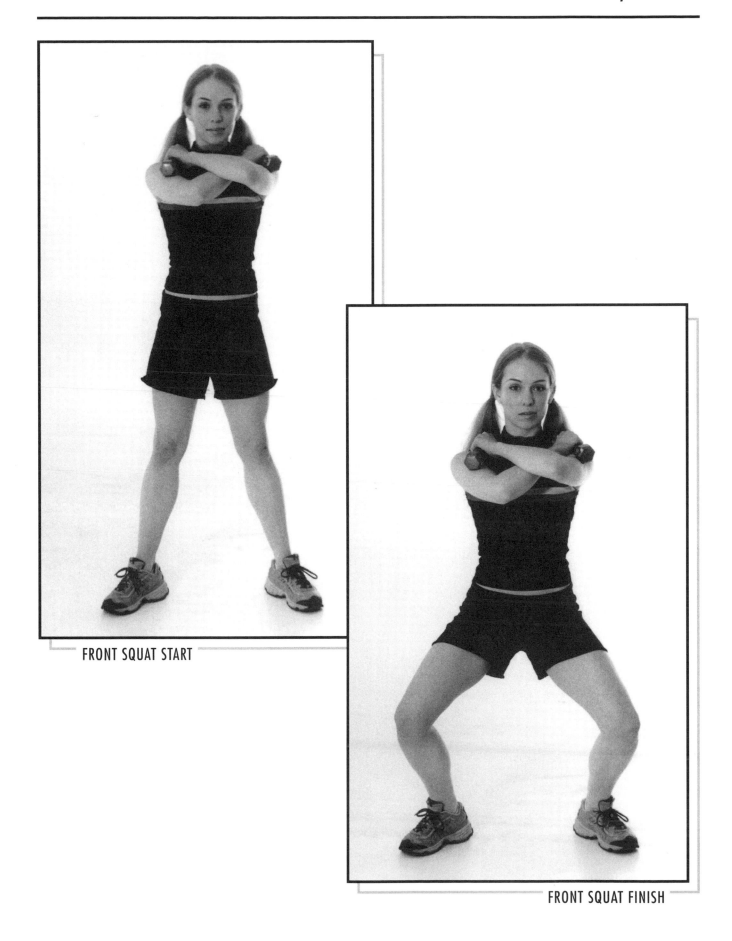

FRONT SQUAT START

FRONT SQUAT FINISH

5. Hack Squat

This exercise tightens, tones, strengthens, and defines the entire front thigh muscle; helps develop and tone the back thigh muscle; and helps remove saddlebags. In addition, it helps strengthen the hip joints, thighbones, and spinal column.

Stance: Stand with your feet a natural width apart. Hold a dumbbell in each hand, behind your back and in line with each buttock and back thigh. Your palms should be facing away from your body.

Movement: Keeping the dumbbells in position as you go, bend your knees until you are at about a forty-five-degree angle or slightly higher—find your comfort zone. Feel the stretch in your front thigh muscles. Flexing your back thigh, front thigh, and hip/butt muscles as you go, and keeping the dumbbells in line with your buttocks and back thighs, return to the start position. Give your front thighs and hip/buttock area an extra-hard flex. Repeat the movement until you have completed your set. Rest for fifteen seconds and move to the next body part, your hips/buttocks.

Tips: Keep your eyes straight ahead and your back straight as you work. Don't hold your breath. Breathe naturally.

<u>**SETS, REPETITIONS, WEIGHTS**</u> (same as page 74, repeated here for review):

Set 1. Light: 12 reps squat + 12 reps lunge + 12 reps leg curl + 12 reps front squat + 12 reps hack squat. Rest 15 seconds.

Set 2. Middle: 10 reps squat + 10 reps lunge + 10 reps leg curl + 10 reps front squat + 10 reps hack squat. Rest 15 seconds.

Set 3. Heaviest: 8 reps squat + 8 reps lunge + 8 reps leg curl + 8 reps front squat + 8 reps hack squat. Rest 15 seconds.

Reminder: See pages 36–37 for tips on heaviness of weights and raising weights.

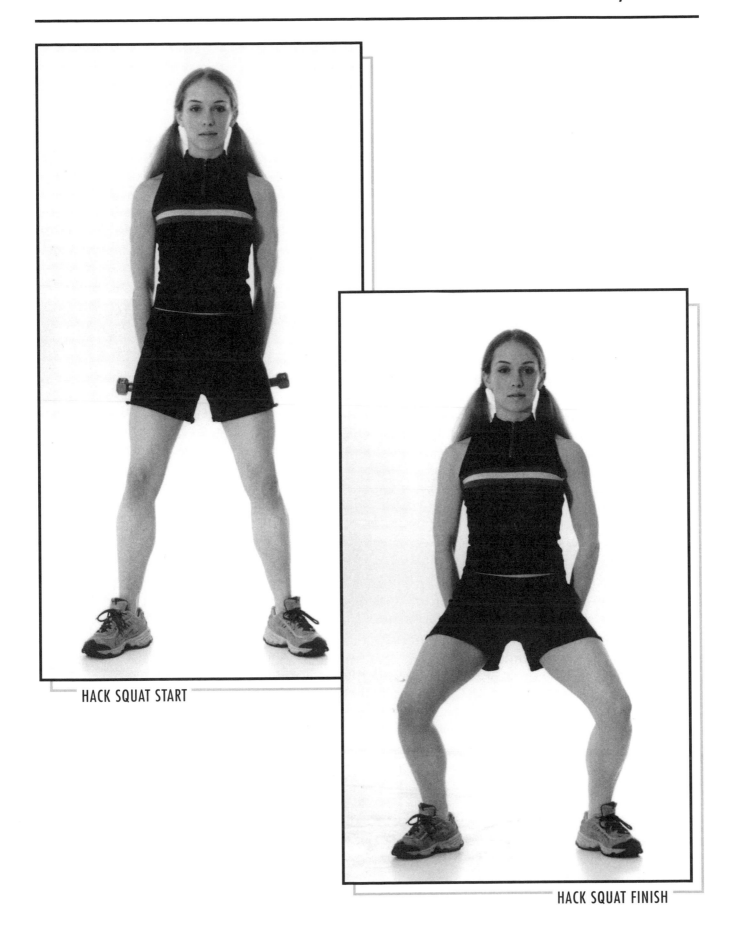

HACK SQUAT START

HACK SQUAT FINISH

Hip/Buttock Routine

1. Lower Butt Side Kick

Slims, firms, shapes, and lifts the entire lower buttock area. In addition, strengthens the hip joints.

Stance: Lie on your side with your lower leg bent back on the floor. Support yourself with your lower elbow and place the palm of that hand on the side of your head. Bring your other arm in front of your chest and place your hand on the floor for support. Bend your upper leg at the knee and raise it about six inches in preparation for the kick. Flex your toes.

Movement: Leading with your heel, kick your upper leg out as far as possible, and flex your buttocks as hard as possible in the final position. Return to the start position. Repeat the movement until you have completed your set. Repeat the set for the other side of your body. Without resting, move to your next hip/buttock exercise, the lower butt curl.

Tips: Be sure to flex your buttocks as hard as possible every time as you extend your working leg. Feel the stretch on the return.

Machines, Etc.: You may substitute any exercise done on a rotary butt machine for this exercise.

SETS, REPETITIONS, WEIGHTS

Set 1. 15 reps lower butt side kick + 15 reps lower butt curl + 15 reps lying butt lift + 15 reps floor feather kick-up + 15 reps straight-leg kick-up. Rest 15 seconds.

Set 2. 15 reps lower butt side kick + 15 reps lower butt curl + 15 reps lying butt lift + 15 reps floor feather kick-up + 15 reps straight-leg kick-up. Rest 15 seconds.

Set 3. 15 reps lower butt side kick + 15 reps lower butt curl + 15 reps lying butt lift + 15 reps floor feather kick-up + 15 reps straight-leg kick-up. Rest 15 seconds.

Reminder: You are now doing fifteen repetitions of every exercise; there are no weights to pyramid.

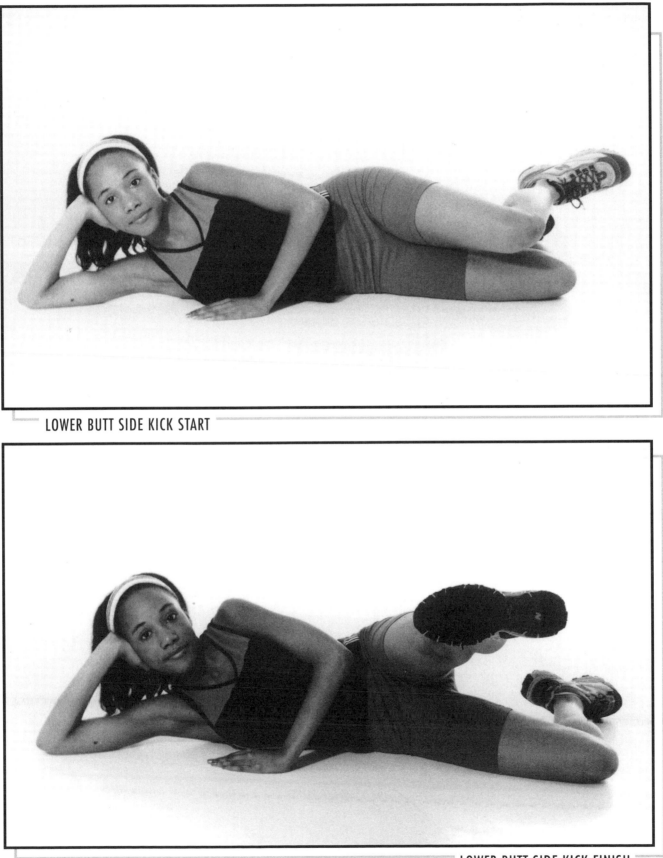

LOWER BUTT SIDE KICK START

LOWER BUTT SIDE KICK FINISH

2. Lower Butt Curl

This exercise tightens, tones, lifts, and shapes the lower butt area and helps reduce saddlebags. In addition, it helps strengthen the hip joints.

Stance: Lie on your side with your lower leg bent back and your upper leg bent and raised about three inches above the lower and slightly forward. Lean on your lower elbow for support and place that hand on the side of your head. Cross your upper arm in front of your chest and place the palm of that hand on the floor for support.

Movement: Bending your knee, curl your upper leg behind you until it's completely straight and you feel a full flex in your working buttock muscle. With full control, return to the start position. Repeat the movement until you have completed your set. Repeat the set for the other side of your body. Without resting, move to your next hip/buttock exercise, the lying butt lift.

Tips: Keep your mind riveted on your working hip/buttock muscle and flex as hard as possible on the return movement. Don't hold your breath. Breathe naturally.

Machines, Etc.: You may perform this exercise on any butt curl machine.

SETS, REPETITIONS, WEIGHTS (same as page 84, repeated here for review):

Set 1. 15 reps lower butt side kick + 15 reps lower butt curl + 15 reps lying butt lift + 15 reps floor feather kick-up + 15 reps straight-leg kick-up. Rest 15 seconds.

Set 2. 15 reps lower butt side kick + 15 reps lower butt curl + 15 reps lying butt lift + 15 reps floor feather kick-up + 15 reps straight-leg kick-up. Rest 15 seconds.

Set 3. 15 reps lower butt side kick + 15 reps lower butt curl + 15 reps lying butt lift + 15 reps floor feather kick-up + 15 reps straight-leg kick-up. Rest 15 seconds.

Reminder: You are now doing fifteen repetitions of every exercise; there are no weights to pyramid.

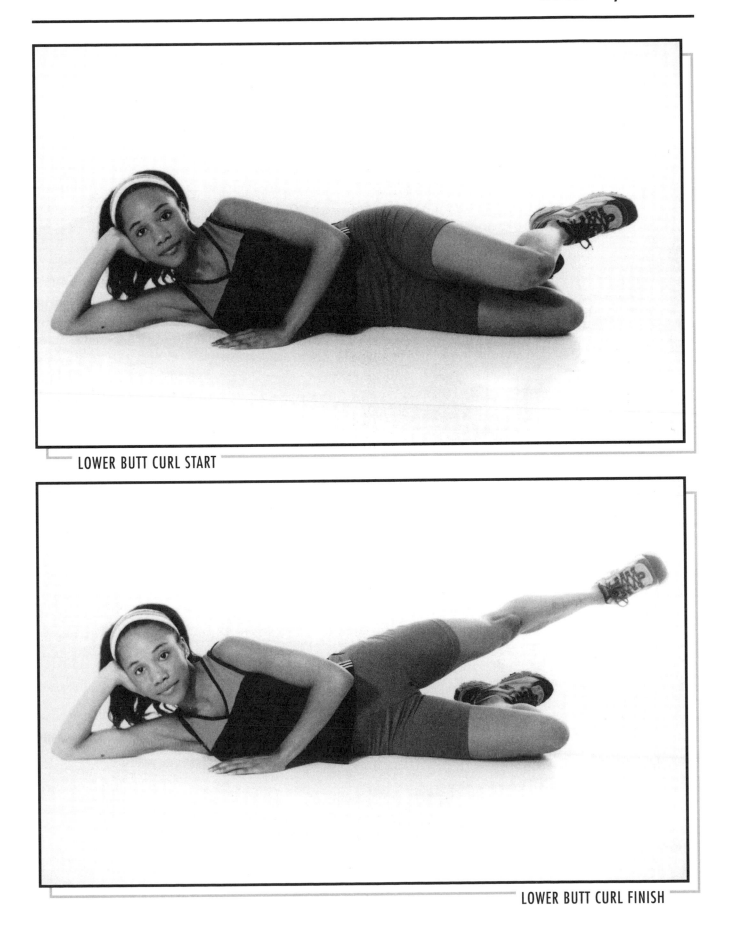

LOWER BUTT CURL START

LOWER BUTT CURL FINISH

3. Lying Butt Lift

This exercise tightens, tones, lifts, and shapes the entire hip/buttock area. It also helps strengthen the lower back and pelvic area.

Stance: Lie on the floor flat on your back with your knees bent and the soles of your feet flat on the floor. Extend your arms out in front of you and place the palms of your hands on the floor, or clasp your hands behind your head.

Movement: Keeping your back and the soles of your feet flat against the floor and squeezing your entire hip/buttock area as hard as possible, raise your hips/buttocks off the floor. (You will be lifting only about three inches.) On the high position, give your hips/buttock area an extra-hard flex and return to the start position. Repeat the movement until you have completed your set. Without resting, move to your next hip/buttock exercise, the floor feather kick-up.

Tips: In order to get the most out of this exercise, you must flex hard on the up movement. Keep your back and the soles of your feet on the floor throughout the movement. Don't hold your breath. Breathe naturally.

Machines, Etc.: You may substitute any exercise done on a hip/buttock machine for this exercise. Set the weight at twenty pounds.

SETS, REPETITIONS, WEIGHTS (same as page 84, repeated here for review):

Set 1. 15 reps lower butt side kick + 15 reps lower butt curl + 15 reps lying butt lift + 15 reps floor feather kick-up + 15 reps straight-leg kick-up. Rest 15 seconds.

Set 2. 15 reps lower butt side kick + 15 reps lower butt curl + 15 reps lying butt lift + 15 reps floor feather kick-up + 15 reps straight-leg kick-up. Rest 15 seconds.

Set 3. 15 reps lower butt side kick + 15 reps lower butt curl + 15 reps lying butt lift + 15 reps floor feather kick-up + 15 reps straight-leg kick-up. Rest 15 seconds.

Reminder: You are now doing fifteen repetitions of every exercise; there are no weights to pyramid.

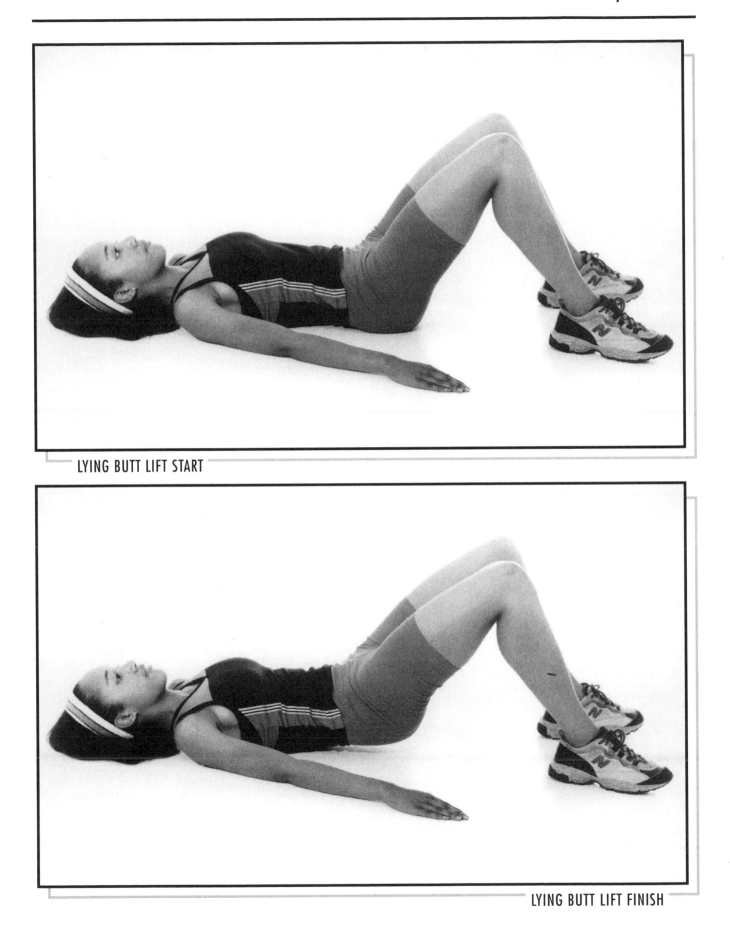

LYING BUTT LIFT START

LYING BUTT LIFT FINISH

4. Floor Feather Kick-Up

This exercise shapes, tightens, tones, and lifts the entire hip/buttock area and helps firm the back thigh muscle. It also helps strengthen the hip joints.

Stance: Get into an all-fours position on the floor.

Movement: Flexing your working foot forward, extend your working leg up and behind you until it is parallel to your body. Your knee should be completely unbent. In this position, flex your working buttock as hard as possible and, in full control, return to the start position. Repeat the movement until you have completed your set. Repeat the set for the other side of your body. Without resting, move to your final thigh exercise, the straight-leg kick-up.

Tips: Use controlled movements at all times—don't swing your leg up and down. Flex hard on the up movement and feel the stretch on the down movement. You may perform this exercise by extending your working leg to a parallel-to-the-floor position instead of a ninety-degree angle.

Machines, Etc.: You may substitute an exercise performed on any hip/buttock machine.

<u>**SETS, REPETITIONS, WEIGHTS**</u> (same as page 84, repeated here for review):

Set 1. 15 reps lower butt side kick + 15 reps lower butt curl + 15 reps lying butt lift + 15 reps floor feather kick-up + 15 reps straight-leg kick-up. Rest 15 seconds.

Set 2. 15 reps lower butt side kick + 15 reps lower butt curl + 15 reps lying butt lift + 15 reps floor feather kick-up + 15 reps straight-leg kick-up. Rest 15 seconds.

Set 3. 15 reps lower butt side kick + 15 reps lower butt curl + 15 reps lying butt lift + 15 reps floor feather kick-up + 15 reps straight-leg kick-up. Rest 15 seconds.

Reminder: You are now doing fifteen repetitions of every exercise; there are no weights to pyramid.

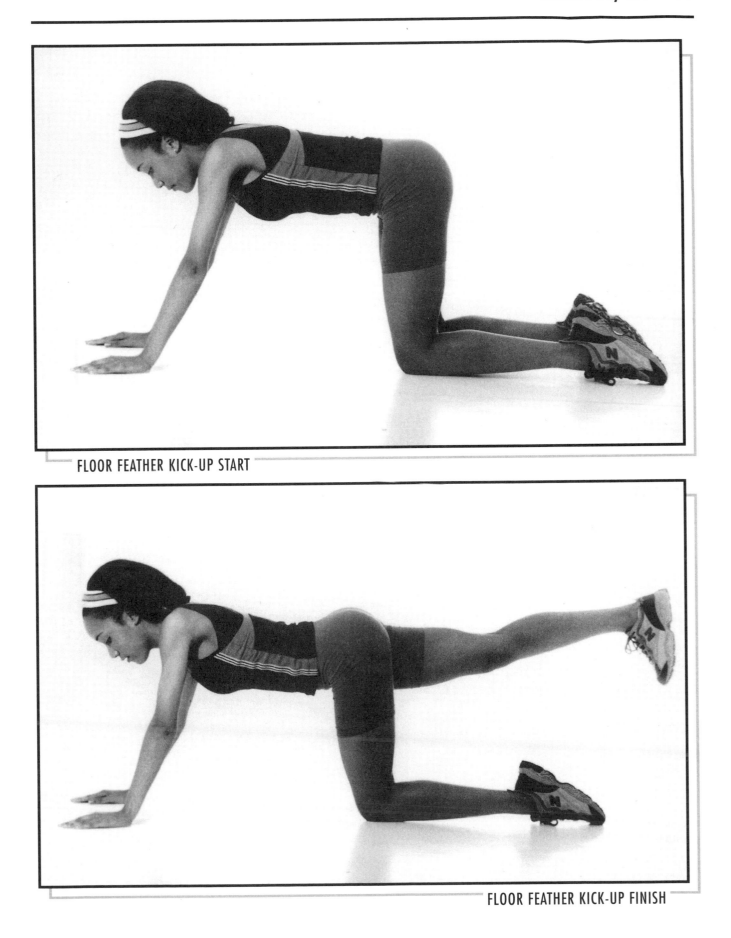

FLOOR FEATHER KICK-UP START

FLOOR FEATHER KICK-UP FINISH

5. Straight-Leg Kick-Up

This exercise tightens, tones, lifts, and shapes the entire buttock area, and helps remove saddlebags. In addition, it helps strengthen the hip joints.

Stance: Get onto all fours on the floor. Extend one leg straight out behind you, in line with your body, and flex the foot of that leg forward.

Movement: Flexing your working buttock as hard as possible as you move, raise your extended leg until it's parallel to your body. Give your working buttock an extra-hard flex and, continuing to keep the pressure on your buttock muscle, return to the start position. Repeat the movement until you have completed your set. Repeat the set for the other side of your body. Rest for fifteen seconds and move to your next body part, the abdominals.

Tips: Extend your leg behind you and keep your foot flexed downward. Make sure you keep your working leg behind your body. Don't hold your breath. Breathe naturally.

Machines, Etc.: You may substitute any exercise done on a hip/buttock machine for this exercise.

SETS, REPETITIONS, WEIGHTS (same as page 84, repeated here for review):

Set 1. 15 reps lower butt side kick + 15 reps lower butt curl + 15 reps lying butt lift + 15 reps floor feather kick-up + 15 reps straight-leg kick-up. Rest 15 seconds.

Set 2. 15 reps lower butt side kick + 15 reps lower butt curl + 15 reps lying butt lift + 15 reps floor feather kick-up + 15 reps straight-leg kick-up. Rest 15 seconds.

Set 3. 15 reps lower butt side kick + 15 reps lower butt curl + 15 reps lying butt lift + 15 reps floor feather kick-up + 15 reps straight-leg kick-up. Rest 15 seconds.

Reminder: You are now doing fifteen repetitions of every exercise; there are no weights to pyramid.

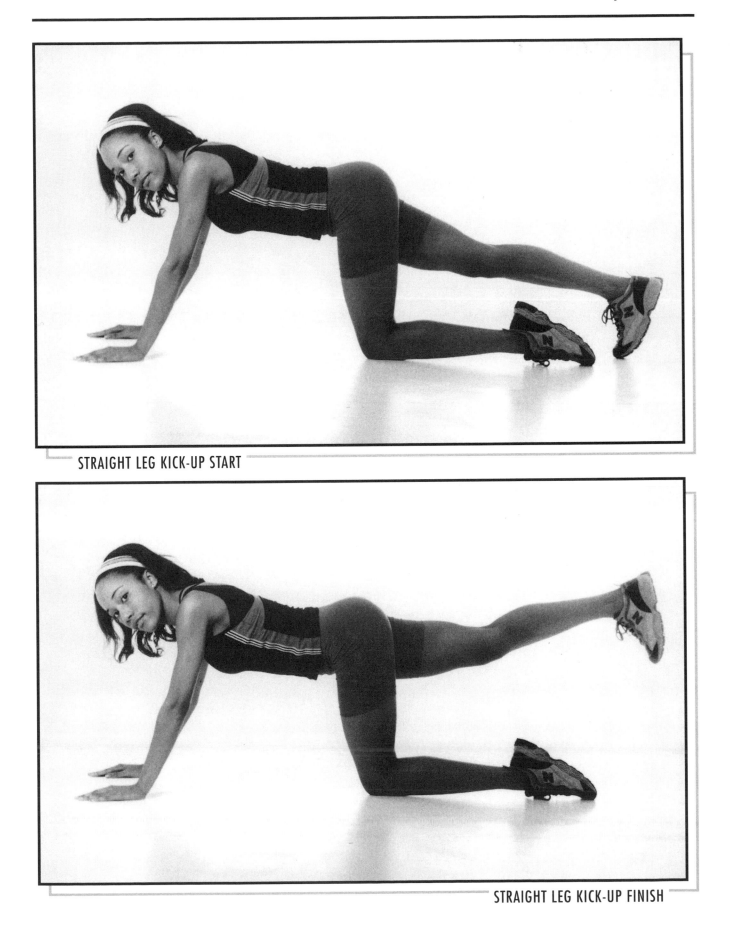

STRAIGHT LEG KICK-UP START

STRAIGHT LEG KICK-UP FINISH

ABDOMINAL ROUTINE

1. Crunch

This exercise develops, strengthens, and defines the upper abdominal muscles, and helps strengthen the spinal column. There are fringe benefits for the lower abdominals.

Stance: Lie on a mat on your back with your knees bent and the soles of your feet on the floor. Place your hands behind your head for support—not for pulling!

Movement: Flexing your abdominal muscles as you go, and in full control, raise your shoulders off the ground. In full control, return to the start position. Repeat the movement until you have completed your set. Without resting, move to your next abdominal exercise, the ceiling sewn lift.

Tips: Don't pull on your neck. Don't jerk up and down or use your arms for momentum. Concentrate on your abdominal muscles as you work. Don't hold your breath. Breathe naturally.

Machines, Etc.: You may perform this exercise on any abdominal crunch machine.

SETS, REPETITIONS, WEIGHTS

Set 1. 15 reps crunch + 15 reps ceiling sewn lift + 15 reps bent-knee sewn lift + 15 reps clamshell crunch + 15 reps ceiling reach crunch. Rest 15 seconds.

Set 2. 15 reps crunch + 15 reps ceiling sewn lift + 15 reps bent-knee sewn lift + 15 reps clamshell crunch + 15 reps ceiling reach crunch. Rest 15 seconds.

Set 3. 15 reps crunch + 15 reps ceiling sewn lift + 15 reps bent-knee sewn lift + 15 reps clamshell crunch + 15 reps ceiling reach crunch. Rest 15 seconds.

Reminder: You are now doing fifteen repetitions of every exercise; there are no weights to pyramid.

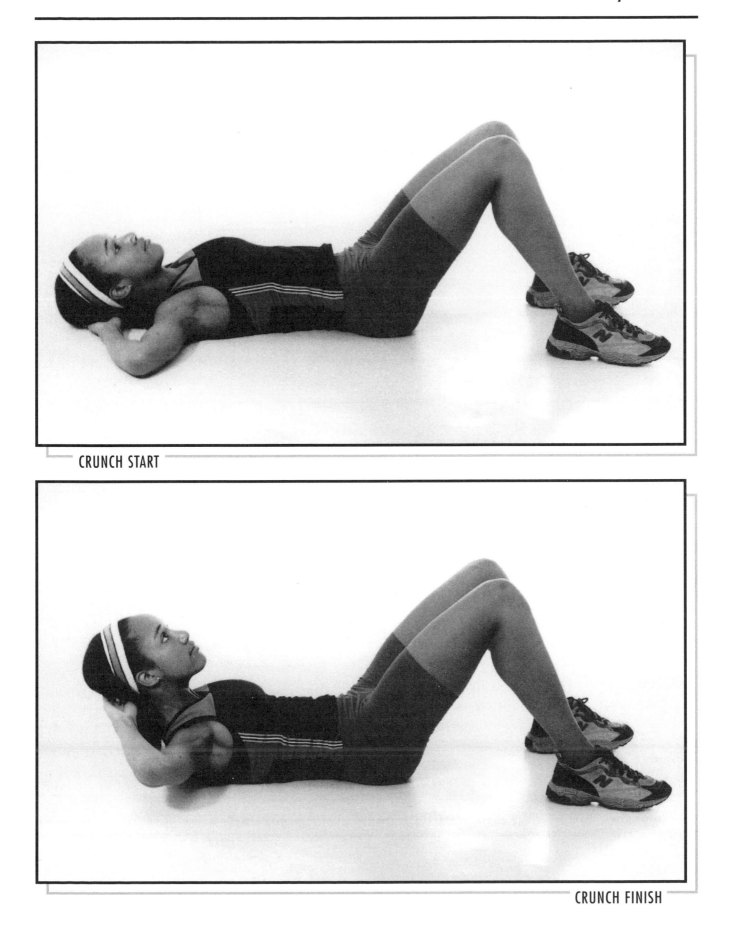

CRUNCH START

CRUNCH FINISH

2. Ceiling Sewn Lift

This exercise tightens, tones, strengthens, and defines the entire lower abdominal area, and helps strengthen the lower back. There are fringe benefits for the upper abdominal area.

Stance:
Lie on the floor and place your hands, fingers interlocked, behind your head. Raise your legs off the floor—extending them fully upward and crossing them at the ankles. Push your back into the floor so that there is no curve in your back.

Movement:
Making believe that your belly button is sewn to the ground, lift your buttocks off the floor about two to three inches while at the same time flexing your lower abdominal muscles as hard as possible. (Remember, you can't go much higher even if you tried. Your belly button is sewn to the ground.) Repeat this movement until you have completed your set. Without resting, move to your next abdominal exercise, the bent-knee sewn lift.

Machines, Etc.:
You may substitute the leg raise demonstrated in my book and video *The Bathing Suit Workout* for this exercise.

SETS, REPETITIONS, WEIGHTS (same as page 94, repeated here for review):

Set 1. 15 reps crunch + 15 reps ceiling sewn lift + 15 reps bent-knee sewn lift + 15 reps clamshell crunch + 15 reps ceiling reach crunch. Rest 15 seconds.

Set 2. 15 reps crunch + 15 reps ceiling sewn lift + 15 reps bent-knee sewn lift + 15 reps clamshell crunch + 15 reps ceiling reach crunch. Rest 15 seconds.

Set 3. 15 reps crunch + 15 reps ceiling sewn lift + 15 reps bent-knee sewn lift + 15 reps clamshell crunch + 15 reps ceiling reach crunch. Rest 15 seconds.

Reminder:
You are now doing fifteen repetitions of every exercise; there are no weights to pyramid.

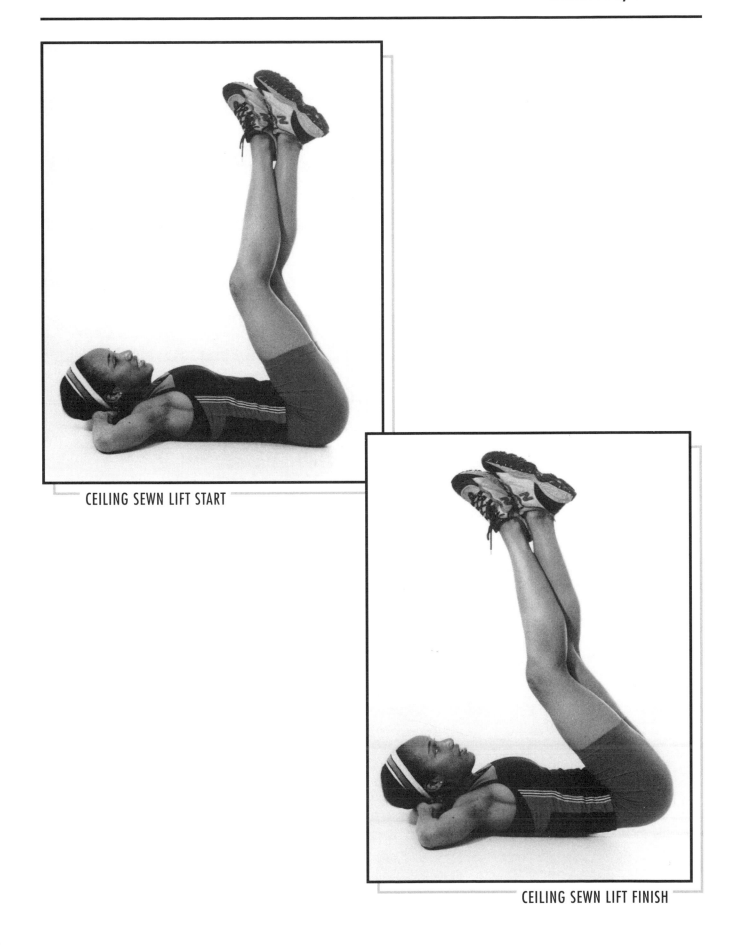

CEILING SEWN LIFT START

CEILING SEWN LIFT FINISH

3. Bent-Knee Sewn Lift

This exercise tightens, tones, strengthens, and defines the entire lower abdominal area, and helps strengthen the lower back. There are fringe benefits for the upper abdominal area.

Stance: Lie on the floor and place your hands behind your head. Raise your legs off the floor—bending your knees and crossing your feet at the ankles. Push your back into the floor so that there is no curve in your back.

Movement: Making believe that your belly button is sewn to the ground, lift your buttocks off the floor about two to three inches while at the same time flexing your lower abdominal muscles as hard as possible. Repeat this movement until you have completed your set. Without resting, move to your next abdominal exercise, the clamshell crunch.

Machines, Etc.: You may substitute the standard knee-in demonstrated in my book or video *The Bathing Suit Workout* for this exercise.

SETS, REPETITIONS, WEIGHTS (same as page 94, repeated here for review):

Set 1. 15 reps crunch + 15 reps ceiling sewn lift + 15 reps bent-knee sewn lift + 15 reps clamshell crunch + 15 reps ceiling reach crunch. Rest 15 seconds.

Set 2. 15 reps crunch + 15 reps ceiling sewn lift + 15 reps bent-knee sewn lift + 15 reps clamshell crunch + 15 reps ceiling reach crunch. Rest 15 seconds.

Set 3. 15 reps crunch + 15 reps ceiling sewn lift + 15 reps bent-knee sewn lift + 15 reps clamshell crunch + 15 reps ceiling reach crunch. Rest 15 seconds.

Reminder: You are now doing fifteen repetitions of every exercise; there are no weights to pyramid.

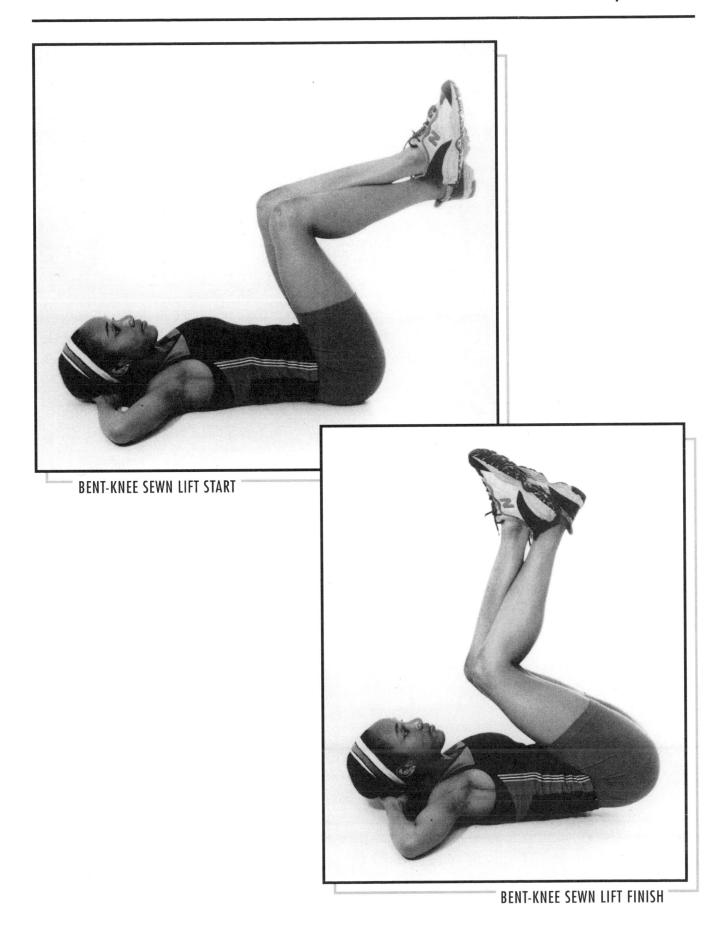

BENT-KNEE SEWN LIFT START

BENT-KNEE SEWN LIFT FINISH

4. Clamshell Crunch

This exercise develops, strengthens, and defines the upper and lower abdominal muscles, and helps strengthen the spinal column.

Stance: Lie on a mat on your back with your knees raised and your feet crossed at the ankles. Place your hands, clasped, behind your head.

Movement: Flexing your entire abdominal area as you go, raise your shoulders and hip/butt area off the ground at the same time. Your back remains on the mat throughout the movement. In full control, return to the start position. Repeat the movement until you have completed your set. Without resting, move to your next abdominal exercise, the ceiling reach crunch.

Tips: Don't pull on your neck. Don't jerk up and down. Concentrate on your abdominal muscles as you work. Don't hold your breath. Breathe naturally.

Machines, Etc.: You may perform this exercise on any abdominal double-crunch machine.

SETS, REPETITIONS, WEIGHTS (same as page 94, repeated here for review):

Set 1. 15 reps crunch + 15 reps ceiling sewn lift + 15 reps bent-knee sewn lift + 15 reps clamshell crunch + 15 reps ceiling reach crunch. Rest 15 seconds.

Set 2. 15 reps crunch + 15 reps ceiling sewn lift + 15 reps bent-knee sewn lift + 15 reps clamshell crunch + 15 reps ceiling reach crunch. Rest 15 seconds.

Set 3. 15 reps crunch + 15 reps ceiling sewn lift + 15 reps bent-knee sewn lift + 15 reps clamshell crunch + 15 reps ceiling reach crunch. Rest 15 seconds.

Reminder: You are now doing fifteen repetitions of every exercise; there are no weights to pyramid.

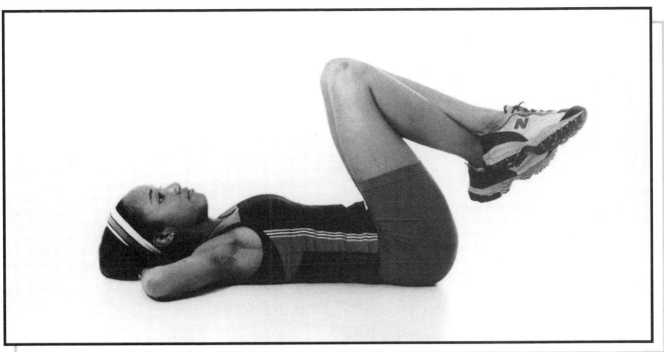

CLAMSHELL CRUNCH START

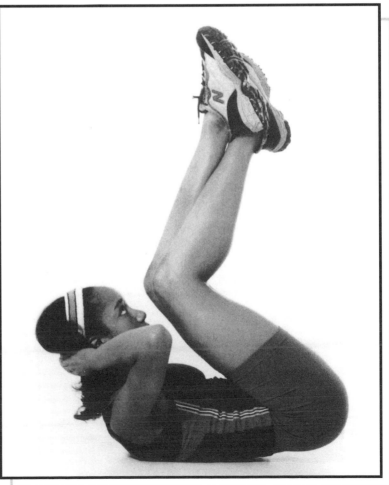

CLAMSHELL CRUNCH FINISH

5. Ceiling Reach Crunch

This exercise develops, strengthens, and defines the upper abdominal muscles, and helps strengthen the spinal column. There are fringe benefits for the lower abdominals.

Stance: Lie on a mat on your back with your legs raised and your knees slightly bent. Cross your feet at the ankles. Extend your arms out at your sides, palms facing your body.

Movement: Flexing your abdominal muscles as you go, in full control raise your shoulders off the ground as you reach toward the ceiling with your arms. (Make believe you are really trying to reach something.) In full control, and keeping the flex on your abdominal muscles, return to the start position. Repeat the movement until you have completed your set. Rest for fifteen seconds and move to your next body part, your calves.

Tips: Don't jerk as you perform the repetitions. Maintain full control. Concentrate on your abdominal muscles as you work. Don't hold your breath. Breathe naturally.

Machines, Etc.: You may perform this exercise on any abdominal crunch machine.

SETS, REPETITIONS, WEIGHTS (same as page 94, repeated here for review):

Set 1. 15 reps crunch + 15 reps ceiling sewn lift + 15 reps bent-knee sewn lift + 15 reps clamshell crunch + 15 reps ceiling reach crunch. Rest 15 seconds.

Set 2. 15 reps crunch + 15 reps ceiling sewn lift + 15 reps bent-knee sewn lift + 15 reps clamshell crunch + 15 reps ceiling reach crunch. Rest 15 seconds.

Set 3. 15 reps crunch + 15 reps ceiling sewn lift + 15 reps bent-knee sewn lift + 15 reps clamshell crunch + 15 reps ceiling reach crunch. Rest 15 seconds.

Reminder: You are now doing fifteen repetitions of every exercise; there are no weights to pyramid.

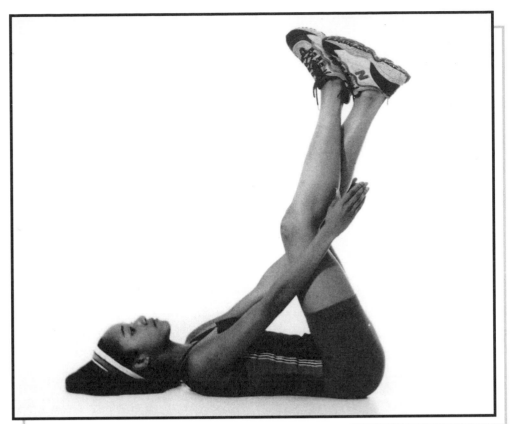

CEILING REACH CRUNCH START

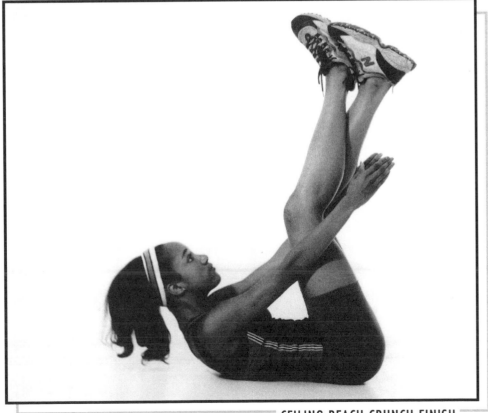

CEILING REACH CRUNCH FINISH

CALF ROUTINE

1–3. Standing-Straight, Angled-Out, Angled-In Toe Raises

These exercises develop, shape, strengthen, and define the entire calf (gastrocnemius and soleus) muscles, and help strengthen the ankle-bones. There are fringe benefits for the shin- and thighbones.

Stance: Stand with a dumbbell in each hand, palms facing your body and your feet a natural width apart. (You can use the back of a chair for balance if you need it—in which case you can do the exercise without weights.) Point your toes very straight ahead for your first fifteen reps, angled out for your second fifteen reps, and angled in for your last fifteen reps. You will be repeating this two more times for three full sets.

Movement: Flexing your calf muscles as you go, rise up on the toes of your feet as high as possible. Give your calf muscles an extra flex and, feeling the stretch in your calf muscles, return to the start position. Without bouncing, and in full control, repeat the movement until you have completed your set. Angle your toes out, then in for your second and third calf exercises. Then repeat the exercise exactly the same way two more times, for your second and third sets.

Tips: You don't need weight for this exercise: Your body can serve as "the weight." If you're using a chair for balance, just let your fingertips graze the chair—don't lean on it. You can also do this exercise one leg at a time.

Machines, Etc.: You may perform this exercise on any standing or seated calf machine. You can also do it seated with a dumbbell on each thigh, placed just above your knee.

SETS, REPETITIONS, WEIGHTS

Set 1. Light: 12 reps standing-straight toe calf raise + 12 reps standing-angled-out toe calf raise + 12 reps standing-angled-in toe calf raise. Rest 15 seconds.

Set 2. Middle: 10 reps standing-straight toe calf raise + 10 reps standing-angled-out toe calf raise + 10 reps standing-angled-in toe calf raise. Rest 15 seconds.

Set 3. Heaviest: 8 reps standing-straight toe calf raise + 8 reps standing-angled-out toe calf raise + 8 reps standing-angled-in toe calf raise.

Reminder: See pages 36–37 for heaviness of weights and raising weights.

Congratulations: You have completed day two, the lower body workout!

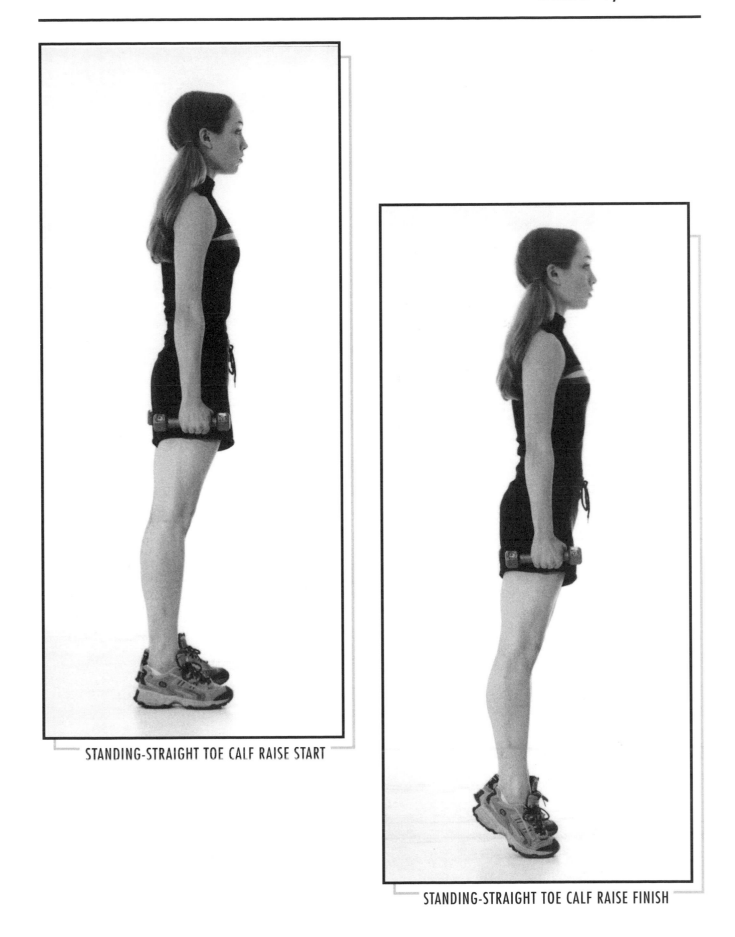

STANDING-STRAIGHT TOE CALF RAISE START

STANDING-STRAIGHT TOE CALF RAISE FINISH

REVIEW OF THE EXERCISES FOUND IN THIS CHAPTER

Thighs

Plié squat
Lunge
Leg curl
Front squat
Hack squat

Hips/Buttocks

Lower butt side kick
Lower butt curl
Lying butt lift
Floor feather kick-up
Straight-leg kick-up

Abdominals

Crunch
Ceiling sewn lift
Bent-knee sewn lift
Clamshell crunch
Ceiling reach crunch

Calves

Standing-straight, toe-out, and toe-in raises

TWENTY-NINE MYTHS AND MISTAKES TO AVOID

One of the first things that will happen to you once you start working out and eating right is that you'll start to hear a lot of talk about shortcuts, new fitness gimmicks, better ways to get in shape, and some outright lies about working out. This chapter is designed to protect you from all of the myths and mistakes out there—and to save you the time and energy you'll waste if you believe the myths and make the mistakes.

1. IF YOU WORK OUT WITH WEIGHTS AND YOU ARE OVERWEIGHT, YOU WILL PUT ON BIG MUSCLES AND LOOK EVEN FATTER THAN YOU ARE.

This is one of the biggest lies ever told. The truth is, muscles take up less space than fat, and help burn fat. What really happens is that you lose fat and go down sizes quickly. Working out with weights replaces fat with lean muscle, which in fact helps burn off even more fat, twenty-four hours a day—even while you're sleeping. After eight to twelve weeks of doing this workout, your metabolism will go up by 15 percent. This means you can eat 15 percent more without getting fat—or lose weight by sticking to your current eating plan!

Why not just diet and wait until you lose the weight to start working out with weights? If you do it this way, once you lose the weight you won't have the right shape. You won't have any definition. Your body won't be hard to the touch. You'll "feel fat," because your body won't be hard like an athlete's. You'll foolishly think you have to lose even more weight, when the real answer is in your workout! So don't you dare wait until you lose the weight. This workout will help you lose the weight faster. And if you're not overweight, the workout will help you get your ideal body.

2. DON'T WORK OUT WITH WEIGHTS BECAUSE ONCE YOU STOP IT ALL TURNS TO FAT.

This is the second biggest lie ever told. It is physically impossible for muscle to turn to fat. It is made up of a completely different substance. The only thing that happens if you stop working out is that the beautiful, defined, sexy muscle you have on your body slowly shrinks back to the size it was before you started. But it takes a while for this to happen— about as long as it took you to get the muscle in the first place. For example, say you worked out for a year and got a prize body. It would take a whole year for your muscles to shrink back to their original size. And the good news is, if you ever start up again, it takes only one-third the time to get back to your toned shape. In other words, in four months you'd be back in shape.

3. YOU CAN'T CHANGE YOUR BODY SHAPE—YOU'RE THE VICTIM OF YOUR DNA. WHATEVER YOUR MOTHER AND GRANDMOTHER GAVE YOU IN YOUR GENETIC POOL IS WHAT YOU'RE STUCK WITH.

This is the third biggest lie ever told. While it is true that your bone structure and a tendency toward a certain body shape are both coded into your DNA, it is *not* true that there's nothing you can do about it. You can re-create your body shape by working out with weights the right way. For example, if I didn't work on my body, it would look almost exactly like my mother's and grandmother's: very wide hips, shapeless legs, sloping shoulders, a big belly, and thin arms. But because I work with weights, I have a perfectly symmetrical body, thighs and all. And guess what? I'm not young! The only thing you can't do by working out with weights, in fact, is get taller—and when you're symmetrical, you'll appear to be the perfect height.

4. THE BEST WAY TO LOSE WEIGHT FAST IS TO GO ON A HIGH-PROTEIN DIET.

Wrong. In fact, this is the best way to lose *water* weight fast and fool yourself into thinking you're losing fat! Also, it's the best way to get much fatter in the long run. Let me explain.

High-protein, low-carbohydrate diets allow you to eat all kinds of fatty protein, including red meats, and hardly any carbohydrates at all. After two weeks of that diet you can lose up to ten pounds—but it's mostly water and some muscle. Why did your body lose all that water?

Carbohydrates help your body hold a balanced amount of water. When you eat a lot of protein at the expense of needed carbohydrates, your body can't hold its required amount of water, and you lose water weight. But the minute you start eating normally (and you must do so eventually—your body will force you to), the pounds return.

When you eat a high-protein, low-carbohydrate diet there are other, more severe consequences. You can't think straight because the missing carbohydrates are what feed your brain. You develop a condition called phosphorous jitters, the result of eating too much protein and too few carbohydrates. You become grouchy and short tempered. You are ready to snap at the slightest provocation. You may get into fights! In addition, you feel weak because carbohydrates are what your body uses as its basic energy source. Some days it will take an act of will even to get up from a chair. Depriving your body of carbohydrates is like trying to drive a car with no gas.

The worst part is that by a week after you go off the diet, you will have gained back at least five pounds, maybe more—and it keeps getting worse after that. Not only do you regain all the water that you lost, but you also gain fat! In fact, you gain and gain. Why? Your body goes into survival mode. You can't stop eating quick-fix carbohydrates such as cookies, doughnuts, candy, cake. Even if you never craved them before, you will now.

Now here comes the real kicker. Once you stop the diet, you are actually softer to the touch—more flabby. Why? When you don't eat enough carbohydrates, your body starts to eat its own muscle in order to have energy or fuel. Since it's muscle that makes your body firm, you feel flabbier. And it gets even worse. Since muscle is the only body material that burns fat 24/7, and you now have less of it, your metabolism goes down and you get fatter just doing the same things you used to do. In other words, you don't burn as much fat as you used to, even in your sleep!

5. LIQUID DIETS ARE A GOOD WAY TO LOSE WEIGHT FAST.

Bad idea. Even if you eat one solid meal a day with the liquid diet, it's not enough. Your body needs solid food on a regular basis; otherwise, once you stop the liquid diet you will eat and eat and eat—it's the survival instinct. In addition, while you're on the diet you will become so obsessed with food that you may even dream about it. Liquid diets help you become obsessed with food. Your life begins to revolve around food, and even when you go off the diet, this continues. It's a bad lesson to teach yourself.

But why does this happen? The human body was created with the urge to chew food for a reason: We need it for our health. Solid food provides our body with bulk and fiber. Bulk and fiber help us eliminate waste and help our bodies prevent all kinds of diseases, cancer among them. In addition, fiber is like a fat vacuum. When you eat fiber, it takes fat along with it when you eliminate your waste materials.

You also gain back the weight if you try a liquid diet. Why? If we are denied chewable food, our bodies find a way to make up for it later by bingeing. Ask your parents if they remember when Oprah, after going on a liquid diet, appeared on TV with a big wagon of fat to show how much weight she lost. Well, a year later she looked twice as fat! She must have been so embarrassed. Later, Oprah learned that she too must work with weights, diet, and aerobics. The bottom line is that you just can't fool Mother Nature. The only way to lose weight and keep it off is to eat a balanced diet and to work out the right way. I'll give you both in this book and you can use it for a lifetime.

6. ALL YOU NEED IS THAT ONE AEROBIC MACHINE THEY'RE ADVERTISING ON TV, OR THAT MARTIAL ARTS VIDEO, AND YOU WILL GET INTO GREAT SHAPE!

Not! Aerobics can never reshape your body—I don't care what kind of machine you are using: a stepper, a glider, any kind of bike, and on and on. I don't care if you kick and punch your way into the next century. The only thing that these will do is give you an aerobic workout and maybe make you a little stronger and better coordinated.

The only way to reshape your body is to work out with mainly free weights and to do it the right way. It took champion bodybuilders years to learn how to reshape the body. I'm giving you all of their secrets here—except you won't bulk up like they do, because you're not going heavy, you're not working out for hours, and you're not, as many of them do, using steroids.

7. YOU CAN GET INTO SHAPE FASTER BY USING MACHINES IN THE FITNESS CENTER OR AT HOME THAN BY USING FREE WEIGHTS (DUMBBELLS).

While some machines are very useful, even bodybuilders do most of their workouts with handheld weights. Why? With dumbbells, you completely control the weights, and you are forced to do all of the work (no cheating). Handheld weights are inexpensive and portable. With one simple set of dumbbells you can exercise nine body parts. You can, as you are doing in this workout, do thirty or more exercises with one simple set of dumbbells. In fact, you could do seventy-five or more, but I don't want to overwhelm you.

With a machine, you can exercise only a few body parts. What about those machines that claim to exercise your entire body at home? It can't work. You have to spend so much time adjusting the apparatus for various exercises that you lose a lot of your workout's efficacy. In addition, those machines don't provide enough different exercises for each body part. You need at least three and sometimes more exercises for a body part. Also, as mentioned above, with dumbbells you are in total control of your movement.

There are some wonderful machines to be used if you want to enhance your workout. You can read about them in the "machines, etc." sections of the exercise instructions.

8. YOU CAN'T GET RID OF CELLULITE!

Not true. Absolutely you can. People like to say, "Cellulite is genetic." While it is true that some people are more inclined to get cellulite, everybody can get rid of it! Cellulite is really only bunched-up fat—looking something like an orange peel—that most people have under the skin. But some people have thinner skin than others, so the bunched-up fat or "cellulite" shows more.

This fat is made up of enlarged fat cells that conglomerate just beneath the surface of the skin, clinging to fibrous tissue for support. If you do the workout prescribed in this book, you will put a smooth sexy muscle under the skin, and this will eventually smooth out any area of cellulite. In addition, of course, you must follow the eating plan to rid your body of excess fat.

9. THE FASTEST WAY TO GET THINNER THIGHS OR TO GET RID OF CELLULITE IS TO USE SPECIAL CREAMS.

Never! The only thing creams do is temporarily remove water from the skin. Your thighs may go down for a day or two, and the cellulite may appear less prominent for a few hours, maybe a day, but the minute you drink any liquid your body recaptures its lost water, your thighs get big again, and the cellulite reappears. The only real value of these creams is to the manufacturer, who is laughing all the way to the bank!

10. YOU CAN REDUCE AND SHAPE YOUR THIGHS, HIPS, AND BUTT BY STAIR-STEPPING.

Not in a million years. The only thing stair-stepping can do is help you burn some extra calories. These machines are fine for your extra aerobic activities, and you do gain a little strength in the hip/butt/thigh area, but that's about it. In order to define, tighten, tone, and shape your thighs, and reshape your hip/butt area, you have to exercise in a specific manner, in designated sets and repetitions, as explained in this book, and you must use weights.

11. YOU CAN'T SPOT-REDUCE.

This is true if you're trying to do it by dieting alone. But it's false if you're using weights to reshape a body part. The fact is, you can totally spot-change any part of your body by working out with weights the right way. Think about it for a minute. Suppose you just exercise your arms using weights, doing biceps curls, hammer curls, concentration curls. What would happen? In time you would have strong, shapely biceps muscles. When you "made a muscle" people would comment, "Wow. You've got some arm there." Would your legs look great just because you worked your biceps? Of course not. Would it have any effect on your stomach? No.

So while we all agree you can't spot-reduce by dieting, you can spot-change by working out with weights. You can do it by targeting specific exercises to specific areas on the body. As you hit the muscle from every angle, you gradually chisel the muscle into the desired form. In the end, you completely reshape it,

But what about dieting? When you consume fewer calories than you burn, you lose weight over your entire body. True, the fat tends to have favorite storage places, such as the stomach, hips, buttocks, and thighs, but it's distributed all over the body. When you diet you lose fat all over; you can't control exactly where the loss will occur.

12. TAKING WATER PILLS CAN KEEP YOU SLIM.

Wrong. The only thing water pills can do is to temporarily reduce water retention. A much better way to keep the water bloat out of your body is to keep your sodium level in check and to drink lots of water. Ironically, drinking lots of water helps flush the excess water out of your body.

13. WORKING OUT WITH WEIGHTS CAN'T HELP YOUR HEART AND LUNGS.

Not true. Working out with weights improves the muscle-to-fat ratio of your body and, in that sense, helps your heart. It *is* true that the best way to improve your heart and lungs is to do aerobic activities, but weight training also helps a lot. And if you eliminate the rests, the workout found in this book is also 100 percent aerobic.

In addition, when you add muscle to your body, you increase your metabolism and burn more fat—your heart benefits that way, too. Finally, weight training makes you stronger and helps increase your aerobic endurance. When you do participate in aerobic activities, then, it's easier than it would be if you'd never worked out with weights.

14. WATCH OUT: IF YOU WORK OUT WITH WEIGHTS, YOU WILL BULK UP AND LOSE YOUR COORDINATION.

Not true at all. If you work out with weights as described in this book, you will put on sleek feminine muscularity. You cannot bulk up. As far as being coordinated, we now know that weight training actually improves balance.

15. IT'S IMPORTANT TO WEIGH AND MEASURE YOURSELF OFTEN TO BE SURE YOU'RE MAKING PROGRESS.

The opposite is true: It's important not to waste time weighing and measuring at all! How will you know you're making progress? Two ways: the mirror and the way your clothing fits and looks. What you see in the mirror is what you get. Scale weight fluctuates daily with water elimination; muscle weighs more than fat but takes up less space. So when you're losing weight, the scale may not show anything, but meanwhile you will be looking and feeling great.

16. AS LONG AS I WORK OUT WITH WEIGHTS ONCE A WEEK I SHOULD GET IN SHAPE.

One or two days a week is better than nothing, but if you want the results I promise, you have to do it four to six times a week. An alternative is to work out your entire body in one day; then you take the next day off. With this plan you could work out two or three days a week. In this book, however, we're using a split routine. For this, six days a week is ideal, but you'll still see results if you work four days a week.

17. IF YOU CAN'T DO THE WHOLE WORKOUT THE FIRST TIME YOU TRY, FORGET IT! YOU'RE A LOSER.

You're not supposed to be able to do the whole workout the first day. You should follow the break-in-gently plan. Easy does it. If necessary, do just a few repetitions of each exercise. In time you'll be doing the entire workout without a problem.

18. IF YOU'RE UNCOORDINATED AND CAN'T DO THE EXERCISES EXACTLY RIGHT, IT'S A WASTE OF TIME.

Not true. As long as you do the workout the best way you can, that's what counts. In time you will improve. It might help you to watch the moves on video. A good place to start is with the *Weight Training Made Easier* video. See page 151 for more information.

19. IF YOU DO THE ENTIRE WORKOUT AND IGNORE THE BREAK-IN-GENTLY PLAN, YOU WILL BE SO SORE YOU WILL HAVE TO GO TO THE HOSPITAL.

Well, you may be very sore, but you won't have to go to the hospital. Still, you may be very very sore and you might even have trouble walking down the stairs. What has happened is that you've awakened muscles that have been neglected perhaps all of your life. Read myth 22 to understand soreness. Then you'll calm down and realize that "this too shall pass." The key is, don't stop working out. If you do that, you'll only have to face the soreness again. Work through the soreness. More about this in myth 21.

20. IF YOU DON'T GET SORE THAT MEANS NOTHING IS HAPPENING, AND YOU'RE WASTING YOUR TIME.

No, not true. As long as you are doing the workout exactly as described in the book, don't worry if you don't get sore. Some people have a higher tolerance for pain than others and may not even notice the soreness. Working out creates microscopic tears and swelling in muscles, tendons, and ligaments, but some people's body makeup may be such that they don't even register what others would call discomfort.

21. IF YOU FEEL SORE, STOP WORKING OUT UNTIL THE SORENESS GOES AWAY.

False. You must keep going the next day and work through the soreness. After working out for about five minutes, you may not even notice the soreness, because the workout serves as a massage to your sore muscles. As the blood circulates through your working muscles, the stiffness goes away. In any case, after a few weeks you won't feel sore at all unless you do something different like raise your weights, work faster, or add more exercises.

22. EXTREME SORENESS MEANS YOU HAVE A DEFINITE INJURY.

Not true. As I noted, soreness is the result of microscopic tears in the muscle fibers, ligaments, and tendons as you work out. They usually occur on the stretch part of the exercise, while the muscle fibers are lengthening, yet at the same time trying to contract in order to deal with the work being required of them. It is slight, temporary internal swelling that causes soreness. If you're sore, you should rejoice. Why? This same tearing-down process will eventually cause the muscle to become denser, stronger, firmer, and also, with this workout, reshaped into a more appealing form.

If you do have an injury, you will experience a sharp and/or continual pain as you try to work out. But if you're in any doubt whatsoever, check with your doctor. The most common weight-training injuries are inflamed tendons (tendinitis), torn ligaments, and tears in the covering of the muscle itself (fascia).

It is very unlikely that you will ever have such an injury with this workout, because you will be lifting very light handheld weights in a controlled manner. When you do increase your weights, you will do so gradually, as explained on page 36–37.

23. IF YOU AREN'T DOING THE WORKOUT IN EXACTLY THE TIME THE BOOK SAYS, SOMETHING'S WRONG.

Not true. You may just move faster or slower than the "average" person. Don't worry about it. Try to keep it moving and don't rush it—but no matter what you do, your pace may be different from other people. I go faster than the time allowed in the book, and so do many other people. But there are also many people who work slower, and take longer. If you're taking *much* longer, you should try to pick up your pace.

24. YOU CAN'T USE A BOOK TO WORK OUT. YOU NEED A VIDEO.

Not true. While it's great to have a video to make sure you're doing the exercises exactly right, I want you to know that literally hundreds of thousands of young ladies have gotten in shape by following my books with photographs and instructions alone. I have their e-mails and their before-and-after photos to prove it—as I will soon have some of yours! But for those of you who want to see most of the exercises in this workout demonstrated, there's good news. As mentioned before, you can get any one of my videos, especially *Weight Training Made Easier*.

25. THIS IS A GIRLS' WORKOUT. GUYS CANNOT DO IT.

False. This workout is exactly the same for men—except they can leave out the hip/butt work, since they don't have childbearing hips. Guys should also start with higher weights—probably five-, eight-, and ten-pounders, but not higher. The workout is very intense. Even guys would have to build up to it. But if a guy wants to use a special workout addressed to him, he could use my men's books, *Top Shape* and *Gut Busters*.

26. YOUNG GIRLS WHO AREN'T OVERWEIGHT DON'T REALLY NEED TO WORK OUT.

Not true. Even if a young lady isn't overweight, she can improve her figure and make it more symmetrical and appealing to the eye. In addition, she can make her body harder and more defined. Finally, many young women think they're fat when they're not because they "feel fat." Working out with weights will cure that once and for all. The body becomes tight as a drum, and the false idea that you have to diet yourself down to bone finally disappears. You realize that it's being in shape that counts, not what the scale says or how thin you are.

In addition, and I know you probably aren't thinking about this, working out with weights is the ideal thing to do now while you're young because you're building your lifetime solid-bone base. If you work out now, chances are that when you get older, you will have double the bone density of anyone else your age—avoiding a ton of health problems.

27. THE OLD SAYING HOLDS TRUE: YOU CAN'T BE TOO RICH OR TOO THIN.

I don't know about the rich part—but for sure, the thin part is absolutely false. You *can* be too thin. In fact, you can be thin and not be in shape. You can be "skinny fat." Just because you diet yourself down to bone does not mean your body looks beautiful. In fact, it will look emaciated and shapeless. Being in shape means having some sexy, shapely muscle on your bones (yes, muscle is attached to bone). Your main emphasis in your fitness plan should be to train for a healthy body that is a delight to the eye. A skin-and-bones body is just the opposite. People secretly want to look away when they see such a body.

28. WORKING OUT WITH WEIGHTS MAY CAUSE YOU TO BECOME OBSESSED WITH YOUR BODY AND ENCOURAGE ANOREXIA.

False. In fact, the opposite is true. When you work out with weights, your body starts to take its ideal shape. Suddenly you see that you're looking better than you ever dreamed—your thighs are defined and shapely, your arms are tight and toned, your shoulders are perfectly sculpted, your back has definition—and you have a V shape, so your waist looks smaller. Your butt is high, tight, and round. For goodness' sake, it was more the workout than the diet in the first place, you realize. You are no longer obsessed with diet. Instead you realize it's a balance—doing the right workout and eating a balanced combination of foods on a daily basis. You learn quickly that the worst thing to do for a beautiful body is to starve it. You see that feeding your muscles healthy, delicious food is the only way to give them the fuel they need to develop and form.

29. WHY WASTE TIME WORKING OUT? YOU CAN GET A PERFECT BODY WITH COSMETIC SURGERY.

Really? Is that why one of the top cosmetic surgeons in the country asked me to help him to get his wife in shape—and why he now recommends my workouts to all of his patients? There's only so much you can do with cosmetic surgery. You can't create hard, shapely, defined legs.

You can't make a high, muscular, tight butt. You can't make shapely, defined shoulders, or lats that make your waist look smaller. About the only thing cosmetic surgery can do is eliminate fat from an area—but if you ever subsequently gain weight, it goes elsewhere and perhaps to a weird place, like your neck. You can enlarge your breasts with cosmetic surgery, but when you work out with weights you can make them look bigger by adding definition and cleavage.

For your information, I'm going to give you a brief rundown on some of the most tempting procedures. Then I'll tell you why I think you shouldn't do them.

Breast Implants

Breast implants do just that—they implant a saline-filled bag under or over your pectoral muscle to permanently enlarge your breasts. It usually takes about four hours; it can be done in a doctor's office but is much better done in a hospital under general anesthesia. But don't do it! You can create a lovely chest area by working out with weights as described in this book. In about ten weeks you will have more definition in your chest, and this will make your breasts appear larger.

Breast implants may cause you problems all your life. You can lose sensation in your breast, and the implants can rupture. Who knows what new thing they're going to find out about the dangers of implants? I'm sure you've heard about the class-action lawsuits involving silicone implants (that's why they're now using saline). But new studies come out all the time. Why take the risk?

In any case, most cosmetic surgeons would agree that getting breast implants as a teen (if your parents were, dare I say it, foolish enough to allow it) is not a good idea. You are not fully developed. Many teenage girls continue to gain breast size all the way through the very late teens.

And who says we need a huge chest anyway? Why not dare to be yourself and work with what Mother Nature gave you? Natural is always better. And should you ever change your mind, at least you'll leave yourself something to look forward to. Why not wait until you're in your late thirties, after you've had your children? (Implants are no fun once you get pregnant—they always have to be redone afterward.)

Keep your life simple. Don't do it!

Liposuction

Liposuction permanently removes fat cells from areas of your body such as your stomach, hips, butt, or thighs by sucking the fat out with small tubes. It usually takes about two hours and can be done under local anesthesia or in a hospital. It takes about two to five weeks to recover.

You don't need it, and here's why. The reason for liposuction is usually a body of fat that a person can't seem to get rid of by dieting. But of course a person can't get rid of a lump of fat if she's not doing the right workout along with following a balanced weight loss plan. If you follow the workout in this book, you'll be able to get rid of the excess fat from your entire body and at the same time tighten, tone, sculpt, and shape the problem body part. Your stomach, hips, butt, and thighs will look a lot better by doing this workout than they would after all the liposuction in the world.

Cosmetic surgery can add to or subtract from your body, but it can't create muscles. Only you can do that, by working out the right way—with weights, as described in this book.

Another thing. Cosmetic surgery can't make you strong, balanced, and athletic. Only working out with weights the right way can do that, too.

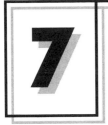

EATING FOR FUN AND FITNESS

I have good news for you. You have to eat in order to lose weight! Yes, it's true. If you don't eat for five hours or more, your body goes into a "slowdown" state and burns fewer calories than it would if you ate the right foods five or six times a day. Why? When you don't eat all day, your body says to itself, "I have to conserve energy. She is going to starve me." So your metabolism slows down and you burn fewer calories doing your normal activities like sitting in a chair and reading a book, or even sleeping. What a waste! You suffer and go hungry and your reward is that you burn less fat.

Ask any medical doctor if you don't believe me. The best way to lose weight is to eat the right foods and portions, and to eat five to six times a day.

DIET IS WHAT YOU EAT ON A DAILY BASIS—TO BUILD YOUR NEW BODY!

The word *diet* really means "what you eat on a daily basis." Most people cringe when they hear the word because they associate it with being deprived. Actually we all diet—only some diet to gain weight! Maybe you've been doing that without realizing it. Now things will change: You'll still be eating lots of delicious foods, only some of them will be different from what you were eating. But don't worry. Once you reach your goal, you'll be able to eat whatever you want all day long, once a week, or something special once a day—and still not gain weight.

YOU CAN'T FOOL MOTHER NATURE: BALANCE IS THE KEY

A balanced diet consists of approximately 15 percent fat, 15 percent protein, and 70 percent carbohydrates. In fact, this diet is very much in line with the USDA food pyramid. Now let's talk a little about the three main food elements you will be consuming: protein, fat, and carbohydrates. When you eat the right amount of these, along with a balanced amount of vitamins and minerals, you lose your excess weight—and in the bargain you become healthy and strong.

How do we lose weight? It's really quite simple. We need to consume fewer calories than we use up in a given day. In other words, we create a calorie deficit so that our bodies have to eat up the excess fat in order to survive. In the following paragraphs you'll find ten rules to healthy, happy weight loss and good health and strength.

RULE 1. CALORIES DO COUNT!

Calories are actually just units of energy in chemical form that come from food. This energy is released to your body whenever you eat. If you eat the exact amount of calories your body needs to sustain its weight, you neither lose nor gain weight. If you eat more calories than your body needs to sustain its weight, your body stores the extra calories as fat—in other words, you gain weight. But if you eat fewer calories than your body needs to sustain itself, you lose stored fat—and of course you lose weight.

There are other things besides eating less food that burn off the stored fat on your body, and thankfully you are doing them: working out with weights. Working with weights puts fat-burning muscle on your body. This muscle increases your metabolism (the rate at which your body burns calories) so that you're burning more fat twenty-four hours a day, even in your sleep. But you must also eat right to help the body to lose all its excess fat. To lose fat, must you totally eliminate fat from the diet? Of course not. But you must control the amount of fat you consume.

RULE 2. FAT IN THE DIET IS NOT A TOTAL ENEMY, BUT YOU MUST LIMIT IT TO 15 TO 20 GRAMS A DAY

Some people like to say, "Well, you can eat as much as you want as long as you eat low-fat or no-fat foods." Not true. A calorie is a calorie is a calorie. However, fat grams have more calories than protein and carbohydrates, because there are nine calories in each gram of fat, while protein and carbohydrates have only four calories. So fat is twice as "fattening" as protein or carbohydrates. In addition, fat uses up little energy in digestion—only 3 percent of its own calories—while protein and carbohydrates use up about 15 to 20 percent of their energy in digestion. When you eat fat, then, *you do get fatter than when you eat protein or carbohydrates.*

Let me explain. Suppose you eat one hundred calories' worth of full-fat ice cream. Ninety-seven of those calories are available for use or to be stored as fat. But if you eat one hundred calories of whole-wheat bread, only eighty of those calories are available to be stored as fat or used.

I can read your mind. You're now thinking, "Okay, so I'll just totally eliminate fat from my diet." No! You can't do that. You will end up eating more calories and actually gaining weight if your fat intake is too low—below 10 percent of your diet. Why? You will feel hungry all the time, and your body will drive you to eat so many calories of no-fat food that you will gain weight.

The truth is, the human body needs some fat in order to be healthy. Did you know that if you didn't have a certain amount of fat, your internal organs would jolt and jut against each other and become damaged? We also need fat for our cell membranes and, yes, our sex organs. Finally, fat is important in helping us make use of calcium and vitamins D, E, A, and K. (More about calcium later.) Having said that, there are some fatty foods that you must totally avoid until you reach your goal!

Fat No-Nos Until You Reach Your Goal

Most people have no trouble finding fat: They just go straight to Burger King and order a Double Whopper or a thick shake. But you don't have to do that. In fact, you'll find plenty of fat in the normal foods you eat. There's even a gram of fat in an apple! For our purposes, we will get most of the fat in our dairy and protein requirements—so no doughnuts or Burger King until you reach your goal. Here's a list of forbidden fatty foods until then:

Fried foods
Butter, margarine, oil, lard—
      any fat except canola or olive oil in very small quantities
Doughnuts or croissants
Chocolate candy
Peanut butter, mayonnaise, fat-containing salad dressings
Avocados or olives
Potato or corn chips
Nuts or seeds
Full-fat ice cream
Sour cream or cream cheese
Cookies or cake
Dairy products with more than 2 percent fat
Pork, veal, bacon
The skin on poultry

Why are these food elements banned until you reach your goal? Take a look at this chart.

Forbidden Food	Fat Grams
Doughnut	12
Croissant	11
Chocolate candy bar	15
5 chocolate sandwich cookies	17
Chocolate milk shake	10
Hot fudge sundae	26
8 ounces potato chips	90
8 ounces tortilla chips	60
8 ounces cheese puff balls	80
8 ounces peanuts	70
Large soft ice cream cone, chocolate dipped	20
Burger King onion rings	15
Burger King french fries	22
Burger King Whopper	36
Burger King Whopper with Cheese	45
McDonald's Egg McMuffin	14
Taco Bell beef burrito	20
Wendy's baked potato with cheese	24
Hot dog	22

Notice that the baked potato has twenty-four grams of fat—but it's not the potato that's the problem. You guessed it, it's the cheese. Without the cheese, there would be only two grams of fat in the potato!

And by the way, you might have heard that you can eat as much fat as you want as long as it's "good" or "unsaturated" fat. Not true. Even though these fats are better for your heart health because they don't clog your arteries, they make you just as fat as any other fat, so you have to limit them in order to lose weight.

Before we leave the subject of fat, you should know a little about cholesterol. It's not fat, but when it accumulates in the arteries it can clog them. It is the cholesterol found in saturated fat that clogs the arteries. Meats such as high-fat beef, pork, lamb and veal; organ meats such as kidney, brain, and liver; poultry skin; lunch meats such as salami, sausage, and bacon; full-fat dairy products; and egg yolks all have the artery-clogging "enemy" cholesterol. You won't have to worry about this kind of cholesterol if you follow the eating plan in this chapter, because you won't be eating enough fat to do any damage whatsoever.

RULE 3. EAT PROTEIN IN BALANCE—TWO TO THREE PORTIONS A DAY

Protein is a very important food element. In fact, you may remember learning in school that proteins are called the "building blocks" of the body. Why? Your muscles, internal organs, skin, hair, nails, and blood are mainly made up of protein. In addition, protein affects the production of the hormones that control your sexual development and your metabolism and growth. Protein also helps regulate the acid–alkaline balance in your blood and tissues, as well as your body's water balance.

Protein consists of twenty-two elements called amino acids. Our bodies can self-produce fourteen of these amino acids, without the help of food or any outside source, but the remaining eight amino acids must be obtained from specific foods. The foods that have these eight essential amino acids are called *complete protein* foods: poultry, fish, milk, milk products, eggs, a combination of rice and beans (this combo together makes up a full protein), and red meat (yes, you can have red meat as long as it's very low in fat).

Your body needs a minimum of about fifty grams of protein a day. Take your actual body weight and divide by two. That is the ideal number of grams of protein for you to eat each day. The tables below list some foods you can use as protein sources. I'm listing the fat grams for your convenience, because, as you know, you will get much of your fat requirement from protein.

Poultry (4 ounces, cooked)*	Grams of Fat	Grams of Protein
Turkey breast	1	34
Turkey drumstick	4.5	33
Turkey thigh	5	31
Chicken breast	4.5	35
Chicken drumstick	6.8	37
Chicken thigh	5	31

*All poultry is without skin and cooked without fat. If the same portions were fried, it would add about fifteen grams of fat to each item! So no frying.

Beef	Grams of Fat	Grams of Protein
90% fat-free beef	11	32
93% fat-free beef	8	32

Fish (4 ounces)	Grams of Fat	Grams of Protein
Mahi-mahi (dolphinfish)	0.8	20.8
Haddock	1	23
Cod	1	26
Sole	1	19
Pike	1	25
Scallops	1	26
Tuna in water	1	34
Squid	1.8	20
Flounder	2.3	34
Red snapper	2.3	26
Sea bass	3.4	25
Halibut	4	31
Trout	4	30

Other Foods	Grams of Fat	Grams of Protein
4 ounces low-fat yogurt	2	6
4 ounces no-fat yogurt	0	7
8 ounces 1% milk	3	8
8 ounces skim milk	1	8
4 ounces (1/2 cup) 1% cottage cheese	1	14
2 tablespoons no-fat cream cheese	0	2
1 slice (ounce) no-fat cheese*	0	6
1 slice (ounce) reduced-fat cheese*	2	6
1/2 cup no-fat ice cream	0	2
3 egg whites	1	9
1/2 cup beans**	1	9
1/2 cup tofu**	6	10
1/2 cup firm tofu**	11	19

*Full-fat cheese has eight to ten grams of fat per ounce (slice). That's just too much fat!
**Vegetarian sources of protein.

What About Pizza?

Now, after having said all of that, I'm going to make an exception and let you eat some full-fat cheese on your pizza. Yes, even when you are dieting. You will have to blot the excess oil off the pizza with a napkin; make sure to keep a fat count and add it in to your daily fat intake if you treat yourself to a slice. Allow five grams of fat for each slice of pizza when you do this. But be sure to blot hard. Figure about two hundred calories per slice. Now let's talk about the food group you'll be eating most.

RULE 4. EAT FIVE TO SEVEN PORTIONS OF LIMITED COMPLEX CARBOHYDRATES AND TWO TO THREE FRUITS A DAY

Carbohydrates supply energy to both your body and your brain. In fact, when your carbohydrate supply is too low, you literally can't think straight, and you become very irritable and weak in the bargain.

The best kind of carbohydrates for gradually released, steady energy are called complex carbohydrates. This group includes breads, crackers, cereals, pastas, potatoes, corn, beans, peas, rice, pretzels, and popcorn (all without butter, of course).

The other kind of carbohydrates, "simple" carbohydrates, release energy much faster, and in the end run out quickly. This group includes all fruits and juice. But you're much better off eating fruit than drinking juice since fruit has bulk and makes you feel less hungry. In addition, the bulk in fruit is fiber—and that helps you in many ways. More about this in a minute.

There are other simple carbohydrates that are processed or "refined." These are not good for you because they create hunger pangs quickly after you eat them. They include sugar in general and all the foods that contain sugar. Be careful because sugar has many names—but it's still sugar. For example, if you read a food label and find sucrose, glucose, dextrose, corn syrup, fructose, maltose, sorbitol, or xylitol—beware, it's really sugar. And guess what? Honey also counts as full sugar. One more thing. Be aware that white flour acts like sugar in the body, so it's much better to eat whole-wheat bread, bagels, and so on.

I've already mentioned that eating sugars makes you feel more hungry very fast—but they can also hinder your body's ability to burn fat because when you eat them, glucose is pumped into your bloodstream at a rapid rate, and your insulin level goes up rapidly. This causes the enzyme that is responsible for pulling fat from your fat cells to be hindered in its work. What happens then is that the fat remains in your cells, and your body is forced to burn carbohydrates in its place.

So where will you get five to seven portions of limited complex car-bohydrates? Here are your simple guidelines.

Breads, Cereals, Grains

1/2 bagel
2 slices whole-wheat bread
1 English muffin
8 low-fat or no-fat crackers
4 rice cakes
1 pita bread
1 ounce cold cereal
2/3 cup hot cereal (after cooking)
2/3 cup pasta, cooked*
2/3 cup rice, cooked
1/2 cup barley, cooked
1 ounce pretzels

Vegetables

1 large baked potato
1 medium sweet potato or yam
1 cup corn
1 large corn on the cob
1/2 cup beans or lentils of any kind (used also as protein)
1 cup peas of any kind
1 cup beets
3 cups popcorn made with no oil

But what if you're still hungry after all this and want to eat more food? Well, there's great news. You can eat as much as you want of the following group—anytime, night or day.

*Cook the pasta until it is firm—not too soft. This prevents it from behaving like a sugar.

RULE 5. EAT SIX OR MORE PORTIONS OF FREE UNLIMITED COMPLEX CARBOHYDRATES TO FILL UP WHEN YOU'RE HUNGRY

You can eat as much as you want of some carbohydrates because they are very low in calories. Your stomach holds only two pounds of food at a time, so you can literally "fill up" on these unlimited carbohydrates if you feel hungry. You can actually feel stuffed without getting fat. Keep in mind that heavy foods make you feel more full than light foods. For example, you'll feel more full eating the free unlimited broccoli, red peppers, and tomatoes than you will just lettuce leaves. The same holds true, by the way, in the limited category. You'll feel more full eating one hundred calories of baked potato (one medium-sized potato) that weighs about six ounces than you will eating two-thirds of a cup of cold cereal—which also has about one hundred calories but weighs only one little ounce. Your stomach simply won't feel as full on the cold cereal. Just some food for thought.

A Minimum of Six Servings a Day

Wait a minute! Why am I saying "minimum of"? Are you actually required to eat them? Yes. In order to keep to this diet, lose your excess body fat, and stay healthy, you must eat the minimum required amount daily. At first you won't want to do it, but in about a week or two you'll become addicted to good eating. Your body will also respond with more energy, better skin tone, and weight loss if you're overweight.

What follows are some sources of complex carbohydrates. A serving equals half a cup of cooked or one cup of raw food.

Unlimited Complex Carbohydrates

Asparagus
Broccoli
Cabbage or Chinese cabbage
Carrots
Cauliflower
Celery
Chicory
Collard greens
Cucumber
Eggplant
Endive
Escarole

Frozen mixed vegetables
Green or yellow beans
Kale
Leeks
Lettuce
Mushrooms
Okra
Onions
Parsnips
Peppers, green or red
Radishes
Rutabagas
Shallots
Spinach
Sprouts
Squash (summer or zucchini)
Tomatoes
Turnips
Vegetable juice, 6 ounces*

The Importance of Fiber

Why do you need fiber? Fiber helps remove fat from your digestive system. When you eliminate fiber (yes, eliminate as in toilet bowl), some of the fat in your digestive system clings to the rough surface of the fiber, which pulls the fat along with it. In this sense, fiber behaves as a "fat vacuum."

Fiber also has many health benefits. The main one for many teenagers is to prevent painful constipation and hemorrhoids—a very common problem in unwitting teens who don't realize that lack of fiber is exactly the reason for this problem. In addition, fiber is known to prevent many health problems that may arise in the future, including colon cancer and other diseases. I know you're not thinking about this now, but it's a wonderful fringe benefit, and you'll be glad later. Now that you're sold, how much do you need and where will you get it?

You need about thirty grams of fiber a day, but don't throw this book across the room! You won't have to think about it at all. Fortunately, you will automatically get that amount and more if you are following this eating plan and eating at least six portions of the unlimited complex car-

*No more than two servings a day. (You need the fiber from the actual vegetables.)

bohydrates and some breads or cereals as is required. How so? For example, there are eight grams of fiber in one cup of broccoli, carrots, or eggplant, and a good amount in all vegetables. There are about five grams of fiber in every piece of fruit you eat. If you're eating cold cereal, you should opt for the high-fiber kind—these usually have about fifteen grams per serving, and you feel more full than you would with the regular cereals. Now let's talk about the last food category, dairy.

RULE 6. EAT TWO TO THREE SERVINGS OF DAIRY EVERY DAY, AND MAKE SURE YOU GET YOUR PROPER AMOUNT OF CALCIUM

Dairy is a very important food category because it provides you with needed calcium. In addition, dairy is very satisfying, and it seems to soothe your stomach and calm you down when you eat it. Don't worry if you're lactose intolerant. Today they have special dairy products of every kind that you can eat.

Dairy Foods

8 ounces skim or 1% milk
8 ounces no-fat or 1% yogurt
4 ounces no-fat or 1% cottage cheese
2 tablespoons no-fat or 1% cream cheese
1 1/2 slices (ounces) low-fat or no-fat cheese
1/2 cup low-fat or no-fat ice cream*

Yes. Believe it or not you are allowed to get your dairy requirement in low-fat ice cream or cheese! Low-fat yogurt, milk, and cream cheese are also wonderful sources of dairy.

Calcium—What Is It, Why Do We Need It, and How Much Do We Need?

Calcium is very important to everyone, especially at your age, because you are literally building a bone base that will last you for the rest of your life.

Calcium is a mineral, and 98 percent of it is stored in your bones. When you don't get enough calcium for your daily needs, your body becomes a thief and starts to steal it from your bones. What happens?

*No more than two or three times a week.

Your bones get thinner and thinner and eventually start breaking. One of the most common problems teenage girls with eating disorders encounter is breaking bones! The eating plan in this chapter includes plenty of calcium to keep your bones healthy, and working out with weights builds bone during the most crucial time of your development.

Even though you and I both know that the real reason you're doing this workout is to look good, you'll be thrilled about this bone-building bonus when you are your grandmother's age. Call it bone in the bank!

Now back to the subject of calcium. How much should you have in your diet? The National Osteoporosis Foundation recommends the following:

Children 1–10 years	800–1,200 mg
Adolescents, 11–24 years	1,200–1,500 mg
Adult women, 25–49 years	1,000 mg

Notice that you are in the category that requires the most! By now you know why—you're building your lifetime bone base. Where will you get your calcium? Mainly from your daily dairy requirement, but also from some vegetables.

Food Sources of Calcium	Serving	Calcium (mg)	Calories	Fat (g)
Yogurt, plain no-fat	1 cup	452	100	0
Yogurt, plain low-fat	1 cup	415	145	4
Yogurt, fruit-flavored low-fat	1 cup	345	230	4
Milk, skim	1 cup	302	80	1
Milk, 1%	1 cup	300	100	3
Ice milk, 3% fat	1 cup	274	225	6
Mozzarella cheese, part-skim	1 ounce	207	80	4
Cottage cheese (1%)	4 ounces	69	80	2
Broccoli, cooked from raw	1 cup	136	40	0
Broccoli, cooked from frozen	1 cup	100	50	0
Collard greens, cooked from raw	1 cup	357	65	0
Turnip greens, cooked from raw	1 cup	252	30	0
Swiss chard	1 cup	128	46	0
Orange juice, calcium-fortified	1 cup	300	104	0
Soybeans, cooked and drained from raw	1 cup	131	235	11
Tofu, soft	4 ounces	108	85	6
Tofu, soft, made with calcium sulfate	4 ounces	145	85	6
Sardines, in tomato sauce with bones	3 ounces	372	151	10.2
Sardines in tomato sauce without bones	3 ounces	165	151	10.2
Lima beans	1/2 cup	48	100	0
Kidney beans	1/2 cup	48	92	0.4

Why did I list calories and fat grams? You'll need this information to incorporate these foods into your eating plan.

Before we leave the subject of calcium, you should know that if you don't get enough vitamin D, your body won't be able to use calcium even if you eat it by the pound. But luckily, even if you're walking to school and are exposed to the sun for fifteen minutes a day, you'll get enough vitamin D from the sun (right through your clothes and even sunblock) to help you use the calcium.

RULE 7. DRINK SIX TO EIGHT GLASSES OF WATER A DAY FOR BETTER SKIN, TO ELIMINATE WATER BLOAT, AND TO PREVENT HUNGER

Drinking water helps improve your skin. Why? It provides hydration, or moisture. But more than that, drinking lots of water prevents water retention. I know lots of people think that if you drink a lot of water, you'll retain it. Actually, the opposite is true. Drinking lots of water helps to flush out the excess sodium in your system, and along with it extra water that may otherwise cause you to look and feel bloated.

But how much salt or sodium should you have in a day and why not eliminate it completely if it causes water retention? Well, you need a certain amount of sodium for good health. In fact, if your body is deprived of sodium, the acid–alkaline balance of your body is disturbed and your muscles begin to cramp. But too much sodium causes bloat. Here's how.

Sodium holds fifty times its own weight in water—so when you consume too much sodium, it holds on to lots of water. This bloats you up, and you feel and look fatter. The bottom line is, balance is the key. Try not to go under fifteen hundred milligrams a day, or over twenty-four hundred.

Don't worry about finding sodium for your requirements. Every food has some—for example, even lettuce has four milligrams a cup. There are 115 milligrams in six ounces of white meat chicken, 602 milligrams in six ounces of flounder, and 48 milligrams in a cantaloupe. If you're short on sodium, you can always eat a pickle (930 milligrams) or some canned soup (on average, 1,000 milligrams a cup). There are five hundred milligrams of sodium in every quarter teaspoon of salt—about two or three shakes of the saltshaker!

One more thing. If you do eat a high-salt diet and retain water, don't worry. It's temporary water bloat. The minute you cut down your sodium, your body will lose its excess water. You can go as low as twelve to fifteen hundred milligrams to get rid of all excess water bloat. It takes about five days to see it all go. Now, let's talk some more about water and why we must drink plenty of it for weight loss and good health.

More than half of your body's weight consists of water. It is the foundation of all of your body fluids, including digestive juices, blood, urine, lymph, and perspiration. It is water that carries the nutrients throughout your body. For this reason, you can't live for very long without it. You could live for a month or more without food, but you could only live a few days without water. Why? Your body loses about three quarts of water a day just by sweating and using the bathroom.

And here's an important point. It's plain old water that cleans your internal organs. Think about it. How do you think your internal organs feel if you only bathe them in dark colas? Give them a break and give them a nice clean shower often during the day.

But why does drinking lots of water prevent hunger? Water is so important to your body that it needs to get it one way or another. Since most foods contain about 70 percent water, if you aren't drinking, your body will drive you to eat, and eat and eat, until it has sucked out the needed amount of water from food. Many times when you think you're hungry, it's not really food your body wants—it's water. So think ahead. Give your body plenty of water—and often.

Exactly how much water should you drink in a given day? At least six to eight glasses, eight ounces each. A good idea is to drink a glass of water as soon as you get up, one before each meal, one with two snacks during the day, and one before bed. You can also drink a glass before and after you do your workout, and anytime during the day.

RULE 8. EAT OFTEN TO KEEP YOUR METABOLISM REVVED UP

If you go more than four hours without eating, your body goes into survival mode and your metabolism slows down. You may think you're losing more weight by not eating for many hours, but actually the opposite is true. You're burning less calories and fat. Let me explain.

Suppose you eat nothing in the morning—you get up at, say, seven o'clock, go to school, and don't eat until lunchtime, one o'clock in the afternoon. You have been up six hours. After about three hours, your body says, "I'd better conserve energy," and your metabolism slows down, from burning, say, ninety calories an hour to fifty calories an hour. So for three hours, until you fed it, your body burned 120 calories less. Now, you could have had two slices of whole-wheat bread in the morning for only eighty calories—and your metabolism would not have slowed down. You would have burned forty more calories, and in the bargain, you wouldn't have felt hungry or weak. (Some people have gotten so used to this deprivation that they don't even notice it). But the bottom line is, you lose more weight by eating small meals often.

So even if you're not hungry, force yourself to eat something starting in the morning and at least every four hours during the day. Actually, you should eat a decent breakfast, because it provides you with energy for the start of your day. (I'll give you some sample meal plans later.)

RULE 9. YOU ARE NOT ON A DIET FOREVER: GO ON THE MAINTENANCE PLAN ONCE YOU REACH YOUR GOAL.

Once you reach your weight goal, you won't have to keep the same exact diet. If you did, you'd keep losing weight until you got too thin. The idea is to enjoy your food life now that you're at your goal. But how can you do that and not gain back the weight?

Here you have a choice. You can either pick one day a week and eat whatever you want all day long on that day, or you can have one treat a day. Let's discuss the details. I'll call them plan A and plan B. With plan A, you get to eat about 20 percent more than you ate when you were dieting—every day. Let's say you ate about eighteen hundred calories a day to lose weight. You can now add three hundred calories a day—for a total of twenty-one hundred—and you won't gain weight. And the good news is, you can eat those calories in *any* food you love. For example, you can have a bag of potato chips one day, a hamburger for lunch the next, and a full-fat chocolate shake the day after that. All of these would be about three hundred to five hundred extra calories. If you find you are gaining weight on this plan it's quite simple. Do the extra snack only every other day.

The other way to go is to use plan B, where you get to eat twenty-one hundred calories extra, or a total of thirty-nine hundred calories in a day. You can have your Double Whopper, chocolate candy, chocolate chip cookies, anything you want. It probably won't add up to more than thirty-nine hundred calories, and in fact, you may well feel sick at the end of the day. Actually, this is a good thing. It is your body telling you it doesn't like to overeat in an unhealthy way.

What happens if you find yourself gaining weight on plan B? Cut your extra eating on this day in half. See how that works. If it doesn't work, try plan A. But what if neither way works and you're gaining weight? The answer is easy. As soon as you gain more than two or three pounds, go back on the eating plan in this chapter until you are again at your goal weight. Then begin to experiment again with plans A and B.

RULE 10. DO YOUR TONING FOR TEENS WORKOUT (AND EXTRA AEROBICS IF YOU HAVE TIME)

This is a combination deal. It's not just the diet, as you well know. It's the workout with the diet, and if you have extra time, you can add in some aerobics to burn off extra fat. See page 152 for suggestions on how to work in the extra aerobics.

Which is most important—the workout, the diet, or the aerobics? Definitely the workout, because it kicks up your metabolism, makes you lose weight, and makes your body tight, toned, and defined. But to see those pretty muscles and that beautiful definition, you must follow the eating plan or your newly formed body won't show through—there will be fat covering it. Aerobics is last only because even if you never did aerobics, but just followed the workout and eating plan, you would still get the body of your dreams. The aerobics help burn off more fat, and are great for your heart and lungs.

REVIEW OF THE DAILY FOOD ALLOWANCE

1. Fifteen to twenty-five grams of fat per day
2. Five to seven portions of limited complex carbohydrates
3. Two or three fruits a day
4. Two to three portions of protein a day
5. At least six servings—and on up to unlimited—complex carbohydrates a day
6. Two to three servings of dairy per day
7. Six to eight glasses of water a day
8. Don't go more than four hours without eating

Okay. Now let me help you by giving you a sample meal plan. The following plan allows exactly the portions described above. You will be consuming about fifteen hundred calories.

A SAMPLE MEAL PLAN

Breakfast

2/3 cup 40% bran flakes cereal	90 calories, 0 grams fat
1 glass 1% milk	100 calories, 2.6 grams fat, 300 mg calcium
1 1/2 cups strawberries	70 calories

Snack

1 cup plain no-fat yogurt	100 calories, 0 grams fat, 452 mg calcium

Lunch

1 cup green beans	52 calories, 0 grams fat, 100 mg calcium
2 slices whole-wheat bread	80 calories, 1 gram fat
1 ounce mozzarella cheese, part-skim	80 calories, 4.5 grams fat, 207 mg calcium
2 medium tomatoes	52 calories, 0 grams fat

Snack

1 large peach	80 calories, 1 gram fat
2 cups lettuce and tomato salad	25 calories, 0 grams fat

Dinner

6 ounces white meat chicken breast	180 calories, 4.5 grams fat
1 cup collard greens, cooked from raw	65 calories, 0 grams fat, 357 mg calcium
1 grapefruit	100 calories, 0 grams fat
1 large baked potato	250 calories, 0 grams fat

Snack

2 ounces pretzels	200 calories, 2 grams fat
1 cup peas and carrots	50 calories, 0 grams fat

Totals:
Calories: 1,459
Fat grams: 16
Calcium: 1,500 mg

Notice that you have followed your required guidelines for protein, dairy, and simple and complex carbohydrates—limited and unlimited.

You had yogurt, mozzarella cheese, and chicken for your protein. You had yogurt and skim milk for your dairy. You had yogurt, 1 percent milk, mozzarella cheese, and collard greens for your calcium requirement. You had bran flakes, whole-wheat bread, a potato, and pretzels for your limited complex carbohydrates; green beans, tomato, lettuce, peas and carrots, cauliflower, and collard greens for your unlimited complex carbohydrates; and strawberries, a peach, and a grapefruit for your fruit.

This is just an example. You can replace the foods and even switch the meals or snacks around—lunch could be breakfast, dinner could be lunch, the snacks all reversed. Anything goes.

BEWARE OF . . .

✳ **Beware of no-fat foods.** They still have calories, which often come from sugar. In any case, calories count—if you eat more than you burn, you gain weight.

✳ **Beware of no-sugar foods.** They still have calories and may have lots of fat.

✳ **Beware of so-called diet foods.** They still have calories and can make you fat. Follow the eating plan in this chapter.

✳ **Beware of health foods that really aren't.** Many foods may seem to be good for your diet but are full of fat and sugar. This category includes granola bars, sunflower seeds, and many foods that claim to have a low percentage of fat. Remember again, it's your total caloric intake at the end of the day that will determine whether or not you lose weight. Follow the eating plan in this chapter.

✳ **Beware of alcohol.** Although you're underage and aren't supposed to be drinking in the first place, I thought I should let you know that alcohol slows down your metabolism so you burn fat at a slower pace. In addition, it can put you off guard so that you eat more. Alcohol itself behaves as a sugar and slows down your ability to specifically burn fat.

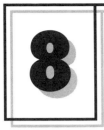

EMERGENCY!

How to Keep to Your Fitness Plan No Matter What

Up to now, it all sounds fine. You have a workout plan and you have an eating plan. They both seem reasonable. But what happens when you're in a position where it seems impossible to stick to your fitness program—to eat right, to do your workout? Let's talk about the eating first.

EATING IN THE SCHOOL CAFETERIA

During any given week, there are a whole variety of foods that may be served for lunch. You may be offered foods such as franks, hamburgers, white or brown meat chicken or turkey, ham, roast beef, corned beef, fish sticks, and tuna or chicken salad. Along with that, as side dishes, there may be, on various days, baked potatoes, mashed potatoes and gravy, french fries, or various other forms of fried potatoes. There may be mixed or plain vegetables of every kind with butter in them, corn on the cob, plain lettuce, tomatoes, cucumbers, beans of various kinds, rice with various sauces, pasta with red or white sauce, and even pizza.

In the dessert area, you may find ice cream, cake, cookies, doughnuts, croissants, muffins of various kinds, ices, Jell-O, yogurt, or fruit. For drinks you will see sodas, juices, and maybe bottled water.

So what can you eat? Having read the diet chapter, you may be able to figure it out for yourself, but just for fun I'll help you. Since nothing fried is allowed, the fish sticks are out (unless you take off the fried coating and blot them hard between three napkins), and obviously the french fries and all forms of fried potatoes are out. Since no fatty things are allowed, no mashed potatoes or gravy (there is also a lot of butter in the mashed potatoes). But what about the buttery vegetables? You can have them, but you must put three or four napkins together and blot them first. Of course the lettuce, tomatoes, and cucumbers are fine, and if they offer raw vegetables or vegetables steamed without butter, great. You can eat corn on the cob, but without butter (blot it off if it's already on). The beans are okay, too, but don't eat more than what looks like two-thirds of a cup.

Always choose poultry over other meats—and choose white meat over dark (that is, the breast over the thigh or leg). Never eat the skin. Simply take it off. But what if only beef is offered? You guessed it. Blot it hard between three napkins to get out the excess fat.

Tuna and chicken salad would be okay—but they're usually made with full-fat mayonnaise, so unless there is no choice, avoid them. The same goes for frankfurters, which usually have lots of fat. You're actually better off blotting the roast beef, corned beef, or hamburger.

Baked potatoes are perfect—just don't put butter or sour cream on them, and if they're already on, dig them off with a spoon. Plain white rice is great, but if it has sauce, it's probably very fatty. I'd rather you eat two slices of bread. Even white bread is better than the rice with sauce, but if they have it, whole-wheat is better. A bagel or English muffin is also fine—if they have them.

Pasta is fine if the sauce is red, not white—the white has too much fat. Again, you can always eat bread in place of the pasta.

Yogurt is great—low-fat or no-fat is best, but you can have full-fat yogurt once in a while with no harm done—even twice a week. Forget ice cream. Jell-O and ices are not a horror, although they are mainly sugar. Try to avoid them. As you well know, all the cake, doughnuts, croissants, and cookies are out. Muffins are iffy. You could have half a bran or corn muffin, but stay away from the rest—too many calories and too much fat. Of course you can have any fruit for lunch. For a drink, don't waste your calories on soda. Drink water—carbonated flavored soda waters are great if they have them.

Bring Your Own Lunch

What can you do if you just don't want to work around the school cafeteria? It's really quite simple. Bring your own lunch. Here are some ideas:

✳ A tuna and low-fat mayonnaise sandwich with lettuce and tomatoes, bottled water, and a piece of fruit
✳ A white meat chicken breast on two slices of whole-wheat bread, carbonated water, and a low-fat yogurt
✳ Eight ounces of cottage cheese and a bagel with tomato and cucumber, and bottled water
✳ A four-ounce can of tuna in water with two slices of whole-wheat bread, bottled water, and a piece of fruit

Be creative. You can bring plastic bags full of cut-up red, green, and yellow peppers, any of the free unlimited complex carbohydrates, cottage cheese, yogurt, a bagel sandwich, pretzels, popcorn, you name it. Just review your food lists in the diet chapter.

FOODS TO BRING WITH YOU OR TO BUY WHEN YOU'RE OUT

Let's talk about what to do if you're going to be out all day and will have no time to stop for food. Unless you bring something with you, you won't eat for, say, seven hours. You already know why this isn't okay. So here are some tips.

First, you can always carry an extra lunch, as above. For example, say you ate breakfast at home, and lunch at school. You know you're going someplace straight from school and won't have time to eat—and you won't get home until 7 P.M. It's *not* okay not to eat from 1 to 7 P.M. You need to snack by four o'clock. You can eat another lunch as a snack if you carry it with you, or you can:

✳ Stop and buy a soft pretzel. This counts as two servings of limited complex carbohydrates.

✳ Stop and buy a low-fat yogurt or cottage cheese.

✳ Bring plastic bags full of cut-up raw vegetables of any kind.

✳ Bring fruit of any kind—but don't eat just the fruit. Eat it with a slice of bread or some vegetables to prevent the rush of sugar and the hunger immediately after.

If you've gotten up late and there's no time for breakfast, no excuses. You can grab a small box of cold cereal (they sell them in serving packs) and eat it on the way to school. Take something to drink with you. Either that or grab a bagel, a container of yogurt, or two slices of whole-wheat bread on your way out the door.

SURVIVAL TECHNIQUES FOR FAST-FOOD EATING

Your first choice is to order chicken. Remove any skin or coatings, and blot it in a napkin. Your next choice is to order a regular burger without cheese and blot it hard in a napkin. If it's a pizza place, you can have two slices of regular or veggie pizza, but blot it hard between napkins. If you have a choice, you can ask for extra tomatoes and less cheese. That helps a lot.

No fries or thick shakes. Order plain bottled water or flavored carbonated water. What about diet soda? True, these are calorie-free and wonderful in that sense, but I worry that too many people are going to have health problems up the road. Make your own decision there.

Beware of salads, because they often have more fat in them than a burger—unless you're choosing vegetables from a salad bar. If they have a salad bar, you can eat, but be careful. Plain tomatoes, lettuce, broccoli, cauliflower, sprouts, radishes, and the like are just fine as long as they're not secretly soaking in some dressing. Eat away with no problem. If they offer baked potatoes, great, but remember, nothing on it! A potato is innocent but cheese, butter, and sour cream are not. You could use spices such as salt and pepper, though.

EATING LUNCH AT YOUR OWN HOME OR A FRIEND'S

If you're at home, you're the boss, so it's easy. Make white meat turkey or chicken sandwiches with tomato and lettuce and mustard or low-fat mayonnaise, or have some pizza (do the blotting!). Another idea is diet pizza—there are various brands available, and some of them are really delicious. As long as they have no more than three hundred calories per serving, you're fine—and some of them even come with pepperoni and other toppings but stay within the three-hundred-calorie limit. Shop around the supermarket. While you're at it, look into the many diet meals they have—pepper steak, chow mein, all kinds of wonderful meals and all under three hundred calories, many only two hundred. These make great lunches. All you do is throw them in the microwave and five minutes later you're eating.

What if you go to a friend's house and all she has is something very forbidden. Well, first use the tricks you already know—blotting and choosing. If that doesn't work, ask for some bread and fruit. You can even eat four slices of whole-wheat bread without doing damage—it's only 180 calories. That and a piece of fruit will get you home just fine. If there's no whole-wheat bread, and there probably isn't, eat two or three slices of white bread. That will work too! But better yet be prepared. If you know your friend never has appropriate foods, bring your own. This is a matter of survival, isn't it? After all, you're trying to accomplish something here, and you may have to fight for it.

COMING HOME FROM SCHOOL STARVING

So you ate your breakfast and lunch—it's only three or four hours since you've eaten. You walk through the door and head straight for the refrigerator and the first thing you see is a dish of leftover stew from last night's dinner. You get a fork and start eating it right from the refrigerator—or maybe you even nuke it for two minutes and then eat. Right? *No.* Mistake. Instead, be prepared. Think ahead. Have stuff waiting for you.

Make a huge tomato, lettuce, cucumber, and pepper salad ahead of time. Have some flavored vinegar and salt and pepper and other spices ready and go to town. Another idea is to have red peppers and cucumbers in the fridge and just cut them up—it takes only thirty seconds.

Or try a can of soup. Any soup is fine as long as it has no more than one hundred calories a serving. Since most cans have two servings, you can eat the whole can—all two hundred calories—and you'll be just fine.

You can also have a melted cheese sandwich! Get a slice of low-fat cheese of any kind and put it on a slice of whole-wheat bread. Sprinkle it with salt and maybe garlic powder and add a tomato. Put it in the microwave for a minute—wow, what a snack! Again, be creative. You don't have to suffer to lose weight.

GOING TO A PARTY WHERE FOOD IS SERVED

Eat pretzels and popcorn (if there's no butter in it) instead of potato chips or nuts. You can eat plenty of the fresh vegetables they usually have—radishes, broccoli, cauliflower, peppers—but don't use the dip that is always so close by. Drink plain or carbonated water—not the soda. Nobody is watching you or expecting you to do anything. You do what's right for you.

DINING OUT AT A RESTAURANT

You may find yourself out for dinner with parents or friends, not sure what to choose from the menu. You already know how to pick and choose using the techniques above, but what do you do when you're confronted with a menu? You look for two things: foods you like and, at the same time, foods that do not break any of the eating rules found in the diet chapter.

For starters, if you don't mind the expense, you can have a jumbo shrimp cocktail. It has very few calories and is delicious. You can even put plenty of the red cocktail sauce on it and of course squeeze the lemon. In addition or instead, you can have a salad—but use only vinegar. Most restaurants have balsamic vinegar—that makes a plain salad taste a lot better.

Another idea for an appetizer, or even for a main dish if you're not in a very hungry mood, is to order soup. In restaurants, chicken with rice, chicken noodle, or vegetable soups are pretty safe. Beware of any of the chowders—they are usually very creamy and fatty.

While you're waiting for your main dish, limit your bread to two slices. Be careful—it's easy to eat the whole basket with butter on it while waiting for dinner. Drink lots of water while you wait. That helps a lot.

As far as a main dish, as you know, you must avoid all fried foods and creamy sauces. Your best bet is baked or broiled chicken or turkey, or fish of any kind with no butter or oil. If it's chicken or turkey, remove the skin. You can have a hamburger if there's nothing else, but again, remember to blot out the excess fat. Yes, I know: People will look at you. So what? And most likely they'll be too caught up in stuffing their faces to care what you do.

Baked potatoes are great and available in most restaurants. You can order any vegetable; most restaurants will serve them without butter or oil if you ask. Pasta is fine with red sauce. Fruit is about the only thing you can have for dessert, and the good news is, most restaurants have delicious fresh fruit combinations. These days, so many people are weight conscious that it isn't as hard as it was years ago to get something delicious and nonfattening.

DINNER WITH PARENTS AT HOME

This can be a big challenge if your parents are unsympathetic to your dieting efforts. But if you let your parents read the introduction to this book, I have a feeling they will help rather than hinder your efforts. You don't have to ask your parents to cook special foods for you—as long as you follow the tricks you learned in this chapter to keep to the basic eating rules, you will do just fine. Of course, if they bake or broil without butter rather than frying, and don't insist that you eat creamy, sugary desserts, your diet life will be that much easier. Maybe you can get your parents to join you in your fitness effort. I've written special books and made specific videos for your mom and dad. You can refer to them in the bibliography. If the whole family works together on a food plan, it's that much easier. But don't think for a minute you can't do it alone. You can. It's your body; nobody is coming along and craning your mouth open and force-feeding you. (At least I hope not.) It is you who raises the spoon or fork to your mouth. It is you and only you who places the food in your mouth, and it is you and you alone who chews the food. So in the end, you have the power, and nobody but you. There may be many things you still don't have power over in your life, but one thing is for sure, you have power over what you put in your mouth.

HOW TO DO YOUR WORKOUT WHEN AWAY ON A TRIP

What can you do when you're away from home and don't have your three sets of dumbbells with you? It's really easy. You just do the movements without the dumbbells—only since you don't have any weights, you do ten repetitions for all three sets, but . . .

Yes. Here's the but. You use what I call "continuous pressure." You flex and use dynamic tension throughout the movement. What you actually do is flex as hard as possible on the contraction part of the movement, and willfully use force on the stretching or elongation part of the exercise. Let me explain.

When you're using weights under normal circumstances, the only time you willfully flex your muscles is during the contraction. For example, when you're doing a biceps curl in the normal fashion, you would flex your biceps muscle as you curl your arm and "make the muscle." At that point you see the bump on your biceps. When you let your arm go back down straight, to the start position, you would control the weight as you lower it—not letting it just drop, but on the other hand, not using any tension or pressure either. But since you're not using weights, you have to make up for it. So you willfully exert tension or pressure on the stretch part of the movement. This is called "dynamic tension." Let me explain further.

Curl your arm upward. Now, as you uncurl your arm, pretend that someone is holding your arm back, trying to prevent you from uncurling it. By force, you are going to make it go down to the straight position. In doing this, you create a force —and this force is called dynamic tension. You create this force yourself, by using your imagination.

Using continual flexing and dynamic tension makes up for the weights and then some. You will quickly find this out if you ever decide to take off a week or two and use this method instead of the weights. When you go back to using weights, even if you were already up to five-, ten-, and fifteen-pound dumbbells, you won't be sore because this method really keeps your muscle fibers alive. It's a whole different feeling than if you had taken off from weights completely for two weeks and then started up again. In such a case, you would be so sore the next day you would hardly be able to walk.

The beauty of this method is all you need is your workout book and yourself—and once you learn the workout, you don't even need the book. You could do this anywhere in the world with no equipment whatsoever!

WORKING OUT WITHOUT A BENCH AND IN LIMITED SPACE

Suppose you don't have a bench and you want to work out. The good news is that for most of the exercises, you don't even need a bench—only the three chest exercises. All the rest are done standing, lying down on the floor, or sitting—and you can sit in a chair just as easily as on a bench.

What can you do for the three exercises that require a bench? You have three choices. You can use a step (the kind used in step aerobics). This handy device can be shoved under a bed when not in use. With it, you have more than enough room to let your elbows descend for the flat bench flye, flat bench press, and cross-bench pullover.

Your next choice is to use a chair and simply tilt it back. In this case you would be doing an incline press or flye—but no matter. The final choice is to simply do it on the floor. In this case you would be losing a little in the range of motion, but it's still a whole lot better than nothing.

OTHER WAYS TO WORK OUT WHEN ON A TRIP

In addition to your weightless workout, you can exercise in many other ways while traveling. First of all, you can take the opportunity to walk a lot—or jog or run if you're so inclined. If you're walking, take off in one direction for thirty minutes, then turn around and go back. You will have walked for an hour and at the same time seen some new sights. If you're running you can cut the time in half—fifteen minutes in each direction. Either way, you've burned about 350 calories. Multiply that by ten and you've lost a pound!

Another idea is to hike the hills. That will up your calorie burning for the same time space to about 450 calories. If you ride a bike outdoors up and down some hills, in half an hour you burn about 350 calories.

Another idea is to jump rope in your room. Boxers do this all the time, for balance and conditioning. You can do it while listening to music or watching TV. This will burn 350 calories in half an hour also.

Waterskiing also burns a good amount of calories—about 270 in thirty minutes. And if you go out dancing, and dance at a fast pace, you burn the same amount of calories in thirty minutes.

If you like sports, you can burn some calories there. Regular downhill skiing burns 220 calories in thirty minutes, and since you're not stopping as much, cross-country skiing burns more—about 320 calories per half hour. Tennis burns about half that! In any case, it's better to be moving and doing something than to be sitting and watching TV or playing video games.

WORKING AROUND AN INJURY

Suppose you injure your arm—even to the point where it's in a cast. Does that stop you from exercising your hips, butt, thighs, stomach, and calves? Of course not. Exercise the body parts that aren't affected by the injury. What if you injure your knee? You can still move your biceps, triceps, chest, shoulders, and back. No matter what the injury, there's usually a way to work on the healthy body parts. Check with your doctor, of course. In addition, your doctor will recommend physical therapy for the injured body part, which almost always involves working out in a moderate, gradual way until you have fully recovered.

If you should sustain an injury, I must tell you that the biggest mistake you could make would be to start using that body part too early. Listen to your doctor. If he or she recommends completely staying off that body part for a given amount of time, pay attention. Why? If you don't take the few weeks now, it will probably cost you a few months, or even more, in the long run.

STAYING IN SHAPE FOR THE REST OF YOUR LIFE

One of the most common questions I get is, "How long do I have to do this?" And my answer is always the same. Forever! And why think of it as a punishment? You probably waste more time on the phone and watching TV than the small time investment of twenty minutes a day—and look at the return you'll get, a beautiful healthy body for the rest of your life.

But some of you will want to go a step farther. In this chapter I'll discuss how to use this plan or other plans (so you won't get bored) to stay in shape for the rest of your life. In addition, I'll talk about adding in your extra aerobics and sports for additional fat burning.

WHAT DO I DO ONCE I'M IN SHAPE?

You have a choice. You can either keep doing this workout forever, four to six days a week with or without the optional extra aerobics, or you can switch workouts—even doing a different one every week.

WHY IT'S A GOOD IDEA TO VARY YOUR WORKOUT

Now that you're in shape and you love this workout, you could actually do it for the rest of your life and stay in shape. But you might not want to work out after a while because you'd be bored to death. Also, your body would get bored—it wouldn't look as good as it could if you did it the favor of switching workouts each week—in a four- to six-week cycle.

Why is it such a good idea to give the body variety? The principle of "muscle confusion" demands it. The idea is to keep your muscles off guard. You do a workout for a week, and just when your muscles are getting ready to relax and take the workout for granted, you surprise them and switch gears. What happens? Your muscles have to be at the top of their game again—they have to perform at a higher level. In short, for the same time investment, you make more progress.

In the following paragraphs, I'm going to explain a possible four- to six-week plan for you. You can use either the book or the video version.

WEEK 1. TONING FOR TEENS

You already know all about this workout. Simply do it four to six days a week, take a day off, and start week two.

WEEK 2. THE TWELVE-MINUTE TOTAL-BODY WORKOUT: DYNAMIC TENSION

This amazing workout does wonders in only twelve minutes a day. How can that be? You use only one simple set of three-pound dumbbells, and do only ten repetitions per set, but you continually flex and use "dynamic tension" on your muscles, so you end up working even harder than when you use regular weights and work out in the normal fashion. When you do this workout, your muscles become very hard. People will comment that "you feel like a rock."

Since the workout is only twelve minutes a day, you don't get a day off, but do it seven days a week. You can use the book *The 12-Minute Total-Body Workout,* or work along with me in the video called *Dynamic Tension: Reshape Your Body in 12 Minutes a Day.*

Dynamic tension is self-imposed force—even on the stretch part of the exercise. In other words, in a normal situation you'd put pressure on your muscle only on the contraction or flexing part of an exercise, but let the muscle relax on the stretch part. With dynamic tension, on the other hand, you apply pressure by resisting as you stretch the muscle. Picture this with a biceps curl. You always flex on the up or contraction movement; in this case, however, on the down movement you make believe someone is holding your arm up and you have to force it down. You apply self-imposed pressure on your muscle as your arm descends to the down position.

You do this with every exercise. It's all clearly explained in the book and video. The beauty of doing this workout the week after your Toning for Teens is that it challenges your muscles in a completely different way. You are working more slowly and deliberately—and doing different exercises.

WEEK 3. DEFINITION

This workout is also available in either book or video form. It is only fifteen minutes a day—but there is a thirty-minute option. It is completely different from the 12-Minute Workout—and like Toning for Teens, but more intense. In Toning for Teens, you do three sets of exercise before you take a rest. With Definition, you do ten sets of exercise before you take a rest. It is more aerobic than Toning for Teens and the 12-Minute Workout; you get exactly what the title says: definition. After doing this workout, your muscles will really show up as clearly delineated and separated from each other. In short, you'll look "ripped."

WEEK 4. WEIGHT TRAINING MADE EASY—OR EASIER!

Having done the balanced Toning for Teens, the slower continual flexing of 12-Minute, and the faster, more grueling Definition, it's time to slow it down a little and do what is called "supersets between body parts." In other words, you do one exercise for, say, abdominals, and one exercise for, say, hips/butt, and keep switching.

The beauty of this workout is that you can keep working out with few or no rests, but you never feel tired because while one body part is working, the other is resting. You feel as if you have had a rest. In addition, because you keep switching, you are able to use heavier weights than in any of the other workouts discussed, and in turn, you can build a solid muscle base—which will further increase your metabolism so you can eat more without getting fat.

This workout takes twenty to forty minutes a day, depending on which option you choose. If you use the book, you can work your way through workout levels one through four. If you opt for the video, which is called *Weight Training Made Easier*, you can advance straight to workout level four as you do the workout with me.

WEEK 5. NONSTOP

Now that you've given your muscles a chance to build, it's time for more definition and fat burning. This workout is 100 percent aerobic. You do not stop to rest at all until you have completed the entire workout. You exercise one half of your body on workout day one—and it only takes twenty minutes. You do the other half on workout day two, and again, it only takes twenty minutes. But since you aren't resting, you're saving more than forty-five minutes of wasted resting time—so the workout is worth an hour.

Here's how it works. On upper body day, you do your first light set of all the exercises for your upper body, and then—without resting—do your second set, with the middle weight, of all the upper body exercises. Finally, and again without resting, you do your last set with your heaviest weight. The exercises are designed and set up so as not to cause exhaustion—in other words, they are placed so that while one body part is working, other body parts have an adequate rest before being asked to work again.

This workout is only in video form, but you can make any of my workouts into a nonstop workout by simply doing them in this fashion. Of course, you'll have to lower your weights and gradually build up because of the intensity of the workout.

TAKING VACATIONS FROM WORKING OUT

Once you're in shape, it's okay to take a week off twice a year—in fact, it's a good idea! What happens when you start up again is that your body actually makes *more* progress. Having been allowed to rest from working with weights, your body is eager to start up again, and says to itself, "I must make up for lost time." You'll find that your muscles actually grow more having rested a week.

Of course you don't have to just vegetate when you take this week off. You should do some aerobics, continue your favorite sport, and in general be active. What if you're sick or have an injury and have to take off longer? Don't worry. Work around it if you have an injury, as discussed on page 147, but if you can't, even if you took a month or more off, don't worry: It only takes one-third the time you took off to get back. I talk about this on page 108.

AEROBICS AND OTHER WAYS TO BURN EXTRA FAT

In addition to weight training, it's a good idea to do some aerobics and participate in various sports. Let's talk about aerobics first. What exactly do I mean by aerobics? An exercise is considered aerobic if it causes your pulse rate to reach between 60 and 85 percent of its capacity, and to stay there for a minimum of twenty minutes. You burn the most fat in the 70 to 75 percent range, so let's do the figuring for that range.

Like I mentioned in Workout 101, you can figure out your 75 percent aerobic range, by subtracting your age from the number 220 and then multiply that by 75 percent. For example, say you are 16 years old. If you do the math, 220 minus 16 equals 204. Now multiply that by 75 percent and you get the number 153. That's quite a high pulse. You're really working. But you don't have to go nearly that high if you don't want to. Even if you get your pulse up to 60 percent—which would be 122—you're okay.

To take your pulse, you can save time by counting for fifteen seconds and multiplying it by four. Find your pulse by placing your pointer and index finger on your wrist or neck.

AEROBIC FAT-BURNING CHART

Aerobic Activity	Calories Burned per 30 Minutes
Running an 8-minute mile (outdoors or on a treadmill)	345
Running a 9-minute mile (outdoors or on a treadmill)	330
Cross-country skiing	330
Swimming	315
Step aerobics	300
Stair-stepping	300
Rope jumping	300
Low-impact aerobics (aerobic dance)	300
Trampoline jumping	245
Race walking	240
Hiking (hills)	240
Jogging at a slow pace (outdoors or on a treadmill)	220
Bicycle riding (stationary or moving at moderate pace)	210
Dancing at a quick pace	180
Walking at a quick pace (outdoors or on a treadmill)	165

You have to realize that these calculations are generalized for people of medium height and weight. If you're very heavy, you'll burn more calories than listed above.

You can do aerobics for ten minutes to an hour—but the ideal amount of time is really twenty to forty minutes, and you can do it three to seven days a week.

If you choose to do aerobics seven days a week, be sure to mix and match—don't do the same thing every day or you may cause a chronic injury. For example, if you run every day you're likely to eventually get shin splints. Pick two or more different activities. You could run one day, ride a bike the next, and use a stair-stepper the next—and keep repeating that cycle. Or you can use any combination. The good news is, your aerobic workout doesn't get in the way of your Toning for Teens workout.

You can do aerobics on any day, whether or not you do your weight-training routine, and you can do it before or after your weight-training workout. I prefer that you do your weight training first, however, only because I know how life is. If you don't do it first, it might not get done—and if there's a choice, you must always put weight training first because you get so much more out of it.

But what if you don't want to vary your aerobic activity? For example, say you just want to run. That's okay—but be sure to give your body at least one day off a week, or in time you may suffer knee, ankle, or other problems.

Break-in-Gently Plan for Aerobics

Suppose you've never done a given aerobic activity. Well, I don't want you to hurt yourself, so please take it easy. If you take the time to break in gently, you can do it forever without a problem. If you rush into it you may get disgusted and quit—or worse, you may be so sore the next day that you won't be able to walk. Worst of all, you may injure yourself. So here's the plan.

Week 1. Three to five minutes
Week 2. Five to seven minutes
Week 3. Seven to ten minutes
Week 4. Ten to fifteen minutes
Week 5. Fifteen to twenty minutes

And if you're going to go that far:

Week 6. Twenty to twenty-five minutes
Week 7. Twenty-five to thirty minutes
Week 8. Thirty to thirty-five minutes
Week 9. Thirty-five to forty minutes
Week 10. Forty to forty-five minutes

ADDITIONAL WAYS TO BURN FAT

If you have a favorite sport, you should take advantage of it as a major fat-burning activity. You can literally work out for hours and never realize you did it. In addition, since you'll be getting stronger from using the workout in this book, it'll be fun to see how much better you are at your sport. This workout will improve your stamina and balance, too.

When you're participating in a favorite sport, the beauty of it is, you're having so much fun that you don't think of it as work—but all the while you *are* working out. You're burning fat and moving those muscles. But remember, your sport is just for additional fat burning. You can't reshape your body with a sport—unless of course you're willing to settle for one pretty forearm (if you're a tennis player), gorgeous legs (if you're a soccer player), or a pretty back (if you're a swimmer). The other thing to remember about a sport is, you can't count on a real aerobic workout because you stop and start a lot. Still, you will burn fat doing a sport. Most sports are played for at least an hour, so the following chart will reflect sixty minutes of steady playing.

Sport	Calories Burned per 60 Minutes
Racquetball	600
Handball	600
Squash	600
In-line skating	600
Basketball	570
Waterskiing	540
Downhill skiing	540
Rowing	540
Canoeing	540
Roller skating	540
Ice skating	540
Tennis (singles)	480
Tennis (doubles)	420
Volleyball	420
Frisbee	420

WAYS TO BURN EXTRA FAT AT HOME

Simply put, you'll burn more fat if you get up and clean your room than you would if you just lay on your bed and watched TV. We do burn fat just lying down, so you would burn about sixty calories in that hour, but if you got up and cleaned your room you would burn at least twice that—and at the same time you'd be getting something done and feel better later (or at least your mom would).

Household Activity	Calories Burned per 30 Minutes
Shoveling snow	375
Washing the car	270
Mowing the lawn	255
Washing the dog	195
Trimming the hedges	150
Mopping the floor	120
Vacuuming	105
Raking	105
Dusting	90

A FINAL NOTE

This is not the end—it's the beginning. It's the start of thinking right about your body and the knowledge that you are in control and can make your body strong, healthy, fit, and a joy to you when you see yourself in the mirror. I know it's not easy to believe it right now, but once you have worked out for a few weeks, you'll see how your whole attitude about your body and your life begins to change for the better. You'll feel empowered and strong, and you'll even start to walk with a different zing! People will notice it—even if they don't mention it.

It's never easy to make changes—but in the end, it pays! You can do it—I know you can. And I'll be right here in your corner, rooting for you and ready to answer you if you e-mail me!

You're off and running. If you want to get more books or videos, see the bibliography. If you have any questions or comments, feel free to e-mail me at jvbody@aol.com. I always answer my mail myself, and I'll be happy to help you. Your mom and dad can e-mail me also. I'd be happy to help them get in shape, too!

RESOURCES

Vedral, Joyce L., Ph.D. *Bone-Building Body-Shaping Workout.* New York: Simon & Schuster, 1999.

——*The Bathing Suit Workout.* New York: Warner Books, 1998.

——*Weight Training Made Easy: From Beginner to Expert in Four Simple Steps.* New York: Warner Books, 1997.

——*Definition: Shape Without Bulk in Fifteen Minutes a Day.* New York: Warner Books, 1995.

——*Top Shape.* New York: Warner Books, 1995.

——*Bottoms Up!* New York: Warner Books, 1993.

——*Gut Busters.* New York: Warner Books, 1992.

——*The Fat-Burning Workout.* New York: Warner Books, 1991.

——*The 12-Minute Total-Body Workout.* New York: Warner Books, 1989.

——*Now or Never.* New York: Warner Books, 1986.

SELF-HELP BOOKS AND AUDIOTAPES

Vedral, Joyce L., Ph.D. *Look In, Look Up—Look Out!! Be the Person You Were Meant to Be.* New York: Warner Books, 1996. (audiotape)

——*Get Rid of Him.* New York: Warner Books, 1993.

VIDEOS AND DVDS

Vedral, Joyce L., Ph.D. *Non Stop.* New York: Joycercize Inc., 2001.

——*Dynamic Tension: Reshape Your Body in 12 Minutes a Day.* New York: Joycercize Inc., 2001.

——*Gut–Love Handle Busters.* New York: Joycercize Inc., 2001.

———*Joyce Explains: Everything You Need to Know about Working Out.* New York: Joycercize Inc., 2001.

———*The Bathing Suit Workout.* New York: Joycercize Inc., 2000.

———*Weight Training Made Easier: Workout Day One.* New York: Joycercize Inc., 2001.

———*Weight Training Made Easier: Workout Day Two.* New York: Joycercize Inc., 2000.

———*Fast Forward: Workout Cycles I and II.* New York: Joycercize Inc., 2000.

———*Fast Forward: Workout Cycle III and Extra Abs.* New York: Joycercize Inc., 2000.

———*Definition: Upper Body Workout.* New York: Joycercize Inc., 2000.

———*Definition: Middle Body Workout.* New York: Joycercize Inc., 2000.

———*Definition: Lower Body Workout.* New York: Joycercize Inc., 2000.

———*The Fat-Burning Workout, Volume I.* New York: Joycercize Inc., 2000.

———*The Fat-Burning Workout, Volume II.* New York: Joycercize Inc., 2000.

The books are found in all stores. The videos, DVDs, and audios are only available through me.

Visit my Web site at www. joycevedral.com.

INDEX

Page numbers of photographs or illustrations appear in italics.

Abdominals or abs (rectus abdominus, external obliques, internal obliques), 30–31
  bent-knee sewn lift, 98, *99*
  ceiling reach crunch, 102, *103*
  ceiling sewn lift, 96, *97*
  clamshell crunch, 100, *101*
  crunch, 94, *95*
  ripped or bear can, 30, 151
  waistline size and, 31
Aerobic exercise, 4, 21
  Break-in-Gently Plan, 154
  cardiovascular benefits, 113
  fat-burning, 136, 153–54
  fat-burning chart, 153
  frequency of workout, 153–54
  machines, 110
  myth: stair-stepping will reduce and shape, 112
  Workout, Week 5: Nonstop, 151–52
Agility, 6, 113
Alcohol, 138
Anaerobic exercise, 21
Anorexia nervosa, 117
Arms
  alternate hammer curl, 56, *57*
  biceps, 28–29
  close bench press, 64, *65*
  concentration curl, 58, *59*
  double-arm kickback, 60, *61*
  one-arm overhead, 62, *63*
  simultaneous curl, 54, *55*
  triceps, 29
Azzariti, George M., xi

Back
  bent lateral, 66, *67*
  double-arm upright row, 70, *71*
  latissimus dorsi, 29
  seated lateral, 68, *69*
  trapezius ("traps"), 29
Balance, 2
Basal metabolism. *See* Metabolism
Bench, flat exercise, 25
  working out without, 145–46
Bodybuilders, female, 3
Body shape or body image, xiv
  balanced musculature or symmetry, xi, 6, 24, 116–17
  baby picture and, 9
  "before" photo, 11–12
  changing, and genetics, 108
  definition, xv
  dissatisfaction with, xv, 1
  ideal, 6, 10, 107
  life's problems and, 10–11
  mind and, 11–13
  put-downs from others, 9–10
  results from weight-training, 6, 23, 113
  self-esteem and, xiv–xv, 9–10
  visualization and preconditioning, 11–12
  weights to shape, vs. aerobics or sports, 4, 110
Bone
  building, with weight-bearing exercises, xi, 116–17
  dairy products as calcium source for, 131–32
  eating disorders and, 132
Breathing during exercise, 21

Calcium
  dietary sources, 131–33
  fat in diet and, 123
  recommended intake, daily, 132
Calories, 122
  aerobic fat-burning chart, 153
  household fat-burning chart, 155–56
  sports fat-burning chart, 154–55
  See also Eating plan
Carbohydrates
  clear thinking and, 109, 127
  complex vs. simple, 127
  energy and, 109
  limited complex, 127
  percent of diet, 121
  simple (sugars), 127
  unlimited complex, 129–30
  water weight and, 109
Cellulite, 111
Chest (pectoralis major, pectorals, or
    "pecs"), 28
  cross-bench pullover, 34, 46, *47*
  dumbbell flye, 34, 44, *45*
  flat press, 34, 42, *43*
Confidence, 5
Control, self, xiv–xv
Cosmetic surgery
  breast implants, 118
  liposuction, 118–19
  weight training vs., 117–18
Cravings: high-protein diets and, 109

Dairy products
  as calcium source, 131–33
  lactose intolerance and, 131
  protein and fat grams in, 126
Definition (Vedral video), 23, 151
Depression: working out and, 6, 15
Diets and dieting
  dangers, starvation and fad, 14, 121
  fiber, need for, 110
  high-protein, 108–9
  liquid, 109–10
  obsessive, xv
  skinny fat and, 2
  spot reduction with, 112
  See also Eating plan
Discipline, 5
  drugs, as destroyers of, 17–18

  self-, xv, 1, 3, 18
  will and, 16–17
  workouts and, xv, 15
Dumbbells, 4–5, 20–21, 24–25
  vs. machines, 110–11, 112
*Dynamic Tension: Reshape Your Body
  in 12 Minutes a Day* (Vedral), 150

Eating plan
  balanced diet, 121–22
  breakfast, 134–35
  bringing food from home or buying
    out, choices, 141
  calories, 122
  carbohydrates, percent daily, 121
  carbohydrates, portions of limited,
    daily, 127–28
  carbohydrates, portions of unlimited,
    free, daily, 129–30
  cautions, 138
  dairy products, 131–33
  density of food and feeling full, 129
  dinner at home, 144
  eating out, 143–44
  fast food and, 12, 123, 141–42
  fat in diet and, 121, 122–23
  favorite foods, 121, 135
  forbidden foods, 124
  frequency of food (min. servings per
    day), 3, 121, 129, 134–35
  ice cream, 131, 131n
  informed choices, xv, 12, 139–44
  juice, 130, 130n
  junk foods and, 12
  lunch, bringing to school, 140–41
  lunch, suggestions for eating at
    home or a friend's, 142
  maintenance plan, 135
  no-nos, 123
  parental help, 13, 144
  parties, eating at, 143
  pizza, 127
  protein, percent of daily intake, 121
  protein, portions a day, 125–26
  review of daily food allowance, 136
  sample meal plan, 136–38
  school cafeteria, 139–40
  snacks, 135
  snacks, after school, 142–43

snacks, preparing ahead of time, 13
training and, 11
unlimited foods, 3, 129–30
water, glasses per day, 133–34
weight loss, necessity of eating
    frequently and, 121
E-mail from teens, xiii–xiv
  address for Joyce Vedral, 156
Emotions, working out and, 14
Empowerment, xiv
Equipment 24–25
  before you begin, 13
  bench (flat exercise), 5, 25
  dumbbells, 4–5, 20–21, 24–25
  machines, 32–33, 110–11, 112
  step, 25
  working out without a bench and in
    limited space, 145–46
Exercise
  aerobic, 4, 21, 22, 110, 136, 151–52
  anaerobic, 21
  defined, 19
  free weights (dumbbells) vs.
    machines, 110–11, 112
  machines, 32–33, 110–11, 112
  movement, 32
  pulse rate, maximum, 21
  repetitions, 32
  speed of movement, 33
  stance, 32
Exercise machines, 32–33
  aerobic, 110
  free weights vs., 110–11
  myth: stair-stepping will reduce and
    shape you, 112

Fast food
  fat grams in, 124
  food choices and, 12, 141–42
Fat, body
  aerobics and, 4, 136, 151–54
  aerobic fat-burning chart, 153–54
  burning, during sleep, 2, 22, 107,
    122
  household fat-burning chart, 155–56
  losing, xi
  sports fat-burning chart, 154–55
  volume and density, vs. muscle, 2, 3,
    107

Fat, dietary
  beef, grams in, 126
  cholesterol and, 124–25
  dairy or soy products, grams in, 126
  digestion and, 122
  fast foods, grams in, 124
  fish, grams in, 126
  forbidden foods, 124
  need for in diet, 123
  no-nos, 123
  percent of diet, 121
  pizza, 127
  poultry, grams in, 125
Fiber, 110, 130–31
  as "fat vacuum," 130
Flex, 20–21

Giant set, 4, 5, 19–20, 33
  chest exercises, example, 34
Gut Busters (Vedral), 116
Guys, workout for, 7, 116
  Gut Busters (Vedral), 116
  Top Shape (Vedral), 116

Health benefits, xi, 14–15
  bone-building, xi, 117–18
  cardiovascular, 113
  fiber and, 130
Hips and buttocks (gluteus maximum,
    gluteus medius, gluteus minimus),
    30
  floor feather kick-up, 90, 91
  lower butt curl, 86, 87
  lower butt side kick, 84, 85
  lying butt lift, 88, 89
  stair-stepping and, 112
  straight-leg kick-up, 92, 92

Injury
  break-in-gently plan, aerobics, 154
  pain and, 115
  tears in fascia, 115
  tendinitis, 115
  torn ligaments, 115
  working around an injury, 147
Intensity, 20

Junk foods, 12. See also Eating plan

Legs
  calf (gastrocnemius and soleus), 31
  front, inner, and back thigh
    (quadriceps, sartorius, abductor,
    and biceps femoris or hamstrings),
    29–30
  front squat, 35, 80, *81*
  hack squat, 35, 82, *83*
  leg curl, 35, 78, *79*
  lunge, 35, 76, *77*
  plié squat, 74, *75*
  straight leg kick-up, 35
  stair-stepping and, 112
  calf raise, standing-angled-in toe,
    standing-angled-out toe,
    standing-straight toe 36, 104, *105*
Liquid diets, 109–10

Metabolism, xi
  alcohol and slowing of, 138
  frequency of eating and, 134–35
  high-protein diets and, 109
  increasing, workout and, 2, 122,
    136, 151
Motivation, 15, 32
  missing workouts and, 16
  psyching yourself, 12–13, 16
Muscles, *26, 27*
  abdominals or abs (rectus
    abdominus, external obliques,
    internal obliques), 30–31
  adductor (inner thigh), 30
  balanced or symmetry, xi, 6, 24
  biceps (upper arm), 28–29
  calf (gastrocnemius and soleus),
    31
  defined ("ripped"), 1, 24, 30
  deltoid (shoulder), 28
  density, 23–24
  fat-burning and, 2, 22, 107, 122
  feminine, xv, 3, 113
  flex, 20–21
  glutes (gluteus maximus, gluteus
    medius, gluteus minimus or hips
    and buttocks), 30
  hamstring (biceps femoris), 30
  hard, toned, xv, 1, 2, 23–24
  isolation exercise, 22
  latissimus dorsi (back), 29

  losing, during inactivity, and
    regaining, 108
  mass, 23
  muscle confusion, 149–50
  muscularity, 23
  pectoralis major, pectorals, or "pecs"
    (chest), 28
  quadriceps or "quads" (rectus
    femoris, vastus lateralis, vastus
    medialis, and vastus intermedius),
    29–30
  recovery time, 22
  results, weight-training, 6, 23, 113
  sartorius (inner thigh), 30
  soreness, 114–15
  stretch, 20, 21
  testosterone and, 3
  trapezius ("traps," back), 29
  triceps (upper arm), 29
  varying routine and, 149–50
  visualizing, 25
  volume and density, vs. fat, 2, 3, 107
Myths
  aerobic machines or martial arts
    video will get you in shape, 110
  big muscles make you look fatter,
    107
  cellulite, you can't get rid of it, 111
  creams can get you thinner thighs
    or eliminate cellulite, 111
  high-protein diets help you lose
    weight fast, 108–9
  if you aren't doing the workout in
    the time the book recommends,
    something's wrong, 115–16
  if you can't complete the whole
    workout, you're a loser, 114
  if you don't get sore, it means
    nothing is happening, 114–15
  if you ignore the break-in gently,
    you'll get so sore . . . , 114
  liquid diets help you lose weight
    fast, 109–10
  machines work better than free
    weights (dumbbells), 110–11
  once you stop exercising, muscle
    turns to fat, 108
  stair-stepping will reduce and shape
    your thighs, hips, and butt, 112

stop working out if you get sore, 115

water pills can keep you slim, 112

weigh and measure yourself often, 113

working out with weights once a week will get you in shape, 113–14

working out with weights will make you bulk up and lose coordination, 113

working out with weights will make you obsessed with your body and encourage anorexia, 117

working out with weights won't help your heart and lungs, 113

you can get a perfect body with cosmetic surgery, 117–19

you can't be too rich or too thin, 117

you can't change body shape, 108

you can't spot-reduce, 112

you can't use a book to work out; you need a video, 116

young girls who aren't overweight, don't need to work out, 116–17

Obesity or overweight teens, xi, xiii. *See also* Weight loss

Pain
  muscle soreness, 114–15
  progress and soreness, 114–15
  sharp and/or continual, injury and, 115
  working through soreness, 114, 115
Phosphorus jitters, 109
Plateaus
  progression of weights, 23, 36–37
  sticking points, 13–14
Posture, 3
Preconditioning, 12
Progression, 23
  raising weights and chart, 36–37
Protein
  beef, 126
  dairy and soy products, 126
  fish, 126
  high-protein diets, 108–9
  percent of diet, 121
  poultry, 125
  servings per day, 125

Psyching yourself, 12–13, 16
Pulse rate, figuring maximum, 21
Pyramid system, 22–23

Recovery time, 22
Repetition, 19
Rest, 20
Routine, 20

Schedule
  break-in-gently plan, aerobics, 154
  first month, breaking in gently, 31
  frequency of workouts, 113–14, 150
  time of day to work out, 15–16
  time, to do workout, 5, 115–16
  workout plans, 38–39
Self-esteem
  body image and, xiv, 9
  negativity, overcoming, 9
  put downs from others, 9–10
  self-discipline and, 18
  source of high, 10
  workout and improved, 3, 5–6, 18
Set, 4, 5, 19
  giant set, 4, 5, 19–20, 33
  superset, 19
Shoulder (deltoid), 28
  alternate front lateral, 50, *51*
  alternate shoulder press, 52, *53*
  side lateral, 48, *49*
Skinny fat, 1, 2, 6, 107, 117
Sodium, 133
Split routine, 22
Sports
  effect on body shape, 4
  fat-burning, 154–55
  fat-burning chart, 155
  weight-training and, 2–3
  working out, while traveling, 146
Spot-reduction, 112
Stamina, 2
Strength, increasing, xi, 2, 6
Stress, reducing, 6, 14–15
Stretch (muscle), repetitions and, 20, 21
Stretching exercises, 32

Target date, 12, 13
Tendinitis, 115

Terms
  aerobic, 21
  "continuous pressure," 145
  definition, 24
  density, 23–24
  diet, 121
  dumbbell, 24–25
  exercise, 19
  flat exercise bench, 25
  flex, 20–21, 145
  giant set, 4, 5, 19–20
  intensity, 20
  muscle confusion, 149
  muscle isolation, 22
  muscle mass, 23
  muscularity, 23
  plateau, 23
  progression, 23
  pyramid system, 22
  repetition, 19
  rest, 20
  routine, 20
  set, 4, 5
  split routine, 22
  stretch, 20, 21
  superset, 19
  weight, 20–21
  workout, 20
Testosterone, 3
Top Shape (Vedral), 116
Training
  attitude and food choices, 11
  effect, xv, 5–6
  12-Minute Total-Body Workout, The
    (Vedral), 150

Underweight and emaciation, xiii
USDA food pyramid, 122

Vedral, Joyce, *xviii*
  background, xiii
  daughter works out with, xv
  Definition (video), 23, 151
  *Dynamic Tension: Reshape Your
    Body in 12 Minutes a Day* (video),
    150
  e-mail letters from teens, xiii–xiv
  e-mailing and address, 7, 156
  Gut Busters (book), 116

Top Shape (book), 116
12-Minute Total-Body Workout, The
  (book), 150
  videos, 23, 33, 150, *see also*
    Resources section
  Web site, 33
  Weight Training Made Easier (video),
    114, 116, 151
  Weight Training Made Easy (book
    and video), 23
Visualization, 11–12, 25

Water
  intake daily, 133
  pills, 112
  skin health and, 133
  weight (fluid retention), 109, 133
Weight, ideal, xi
Weight loss
  aerobic exercise, 4, 21, 136, 151–52
  eating, necessity of and, 121
  eating plan and, 3–4, 121–38
  aerobic fat-burning chart, 153–54
  burning fat during sleep, 2, 22, 107,
    122
  household activities, fat-burning,
    155–56
  high-protein diets, 108–9
  maintenance plan, 135
  muscle-building and dress size
    reduction, 2, 6, 13
  obsession with, xiii
  sports and fat-burning chart, 154–55
  workout with weights, xi, 2, 6, 22
  See also Eating plan
Weight Training Made Easier (Vedral,
  video), 114, 116, 151
Weight Training Made Easy (Vedral,
  book and video), 23
Workout Day One (upper body), 34,
  41
  alternate front lateral, 50, *51*
  alternate hammer curl, 56, *57*
  alternate shoulder press, 52, *53*
  bent lateral, 66, *67*
  close bench press, 64, *65*
  concentration curl, 58, *59*
  cross-bench pullover, 46, *47*
  double-arm kickback, 60, *61*

double-arm upright row, 70, *71*

dumbbell flye, 44, *45*

flat press, 42, *43*

one-arm overhead, 62, *63*

review of exercises, 72

seated lateral, 68, *69*

side lateral, 48, *49*

simultaneous curl, 54, *55*

Workout Day Two (lower body),
  35–36, 73

bent-knee sewn lift, 98, *99*

calf raise, standing-angled-in toe,
  standing-angled-out toe,
  standing-straight toe 36, 104, *105*

ceiling reach crunch, 102, *103*

ceiling sewn lift, 96, *97*

clamshell crunch, 100, *101*

crunch, 94, *95*

floor feather kick-up, 90, *91*

front squat, 80, *81*

hack squat, 82, *83*

leg curl, 78, *79*

lower butt curl, 86, *87*

lower butt side kick, 84, *85*

lunge, 76, *77*

lying butt lift, 88, *89*

plié squat, 74, *75*

review of exercises, 106

straight-leg kick-up, 92, *92*

Workout plans (schedules), 38–39

Workout, Week 1: Toning for Teens

abdominal routine, 94, *95*, 96, *97*,
  98, *99*, 100, *101*, 102, *103*

antidepressant effect of, 6, 15

back exercises, 66, *67*, 68, *69*, 70, *71*

basal metabolism, increasing, xi, 2,
  122, 136, 151

before you start, 7, 11–13

benefits, 6

body fat, losing, xi

body shaping and, 4, 23

bone building and, xi, 116–17

breaking in gently, 31, 114

calf exercises, 36

chest routine, 34, 42, *43*, 44, *45*, 46,
  47

coordination and, 114

Day One, *see* Workout Day One

Day Two, *see* Workout Day Two

different weights for different
  exercises, 37–38

frequency of workouts, 113–14, 150

giant set, 4, 5, 19–20, 33

guys, modifying workout, 7, 116

as habit, 17

hip/butt exercises, 35–36, 84, *85*, 86,
  87, 88, *89*, 90, *91*, 92, *93*

lower body, 35–36

mood and, 14

muscle soreness, dealing with,
  114–15

raising weights as you get stronger,
  36–37, 151

results, seeing, 6, 23, 113

shoulder routine, 48, *49*, 50, *51*, 52,
  53

strength-building, xi

stress, reducing, 6, 14–15

thigh exercises, 35, 74, *75*, 76, *77*,
  78, *79*, 80, *81*, 82, *83*

time of day to work out, 15–16

time, length of, to do workout, 5,
  115–16

traveling, working out during, 145,
  146

varying routine, 149–52

what to expect from, 2–3

working out without a bench and in
  limited space, 145–46

Workout, Week 2, Twelve-Minute
  Total-Body Workout: Dynamic
  Tension, 150

Workout, Week 3: Definition, 151

Workout, Week 4: Weight Training
  Made Easy—or Easier, 151

Workout, Week 5: Nonstop, 151–52

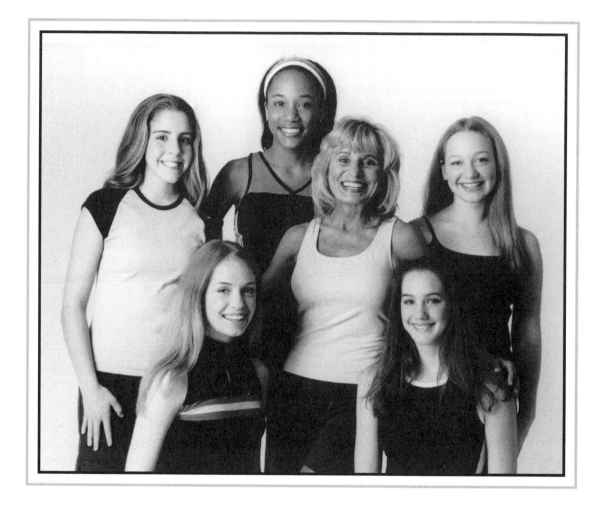

ABOUT THE AUTHOR

Joyce Vedral is a number one *New York Times, USA Today,* and *Publishers Weekly* best-selling fitness author whose books and videos have sold more than three million copies. She is a certified personal trainer, accredited by the ISSA (International Sports Sciences Association). Joyce is also a Ph.D. in English literature (New York University) and has applied her research abilities to the fitness world, where she met and trained with the Father of Fitness, Joe Weider—publisher of *Muscle and Fitness, Shape,* and *Sports Fitness* magazines. Joe gives Joyce's workouts his unqualified seal of approval! Her frequent appearances on the talk show circuit have made her a household name as a fitness expert. Joyce is a sought-after lecturer and fitness instructor. She also taught teenagers at the high school level for twenty-five years.

Joyce says: "After getting fatter every year despite dieting and working out hours a day, I was ashamed to stand in front of my class (I was an English teacher). I did the research and soon realized that champion bodybuilders had the secrets to body shaping. Why reinvent the wheel? I applied the principles to myself, modifying them to get feminine muscularity, and in a matter of twelve weeks my body was transformed." Warner Books became very excited and began publishing Joyce's workouts, which ended up in video—and the rest is history.

Joyce says: "If I can do it, you can do it, too. I didn't even pick up a weight until I was thirty-nine—and looked better than ever in my life in a matter of months." (Go to Joyce's Web site and see her before-and-after photos at www.joycevedral.com.) Now, at fifty-seven, Joyce has the bones and body of a twenty-five-year-old! She says, "The key is to do it—like brushing your teeth or taking a shower. You don't have to get a thrill out of it, just do it." Joyce answers e-mail personally because she says, "I know how it feels to be alone."